DETECTION AND PREVENTION OF ADVERSE DRUG EVENTS

Studies in Health Technology and Informatics

This book series was started in 1990 to promote research conducted under the auspices of the EC programmes' Advanced Informatics in Medicine (AIM) and Biomedical and Health Research (BHR) bioengineering branch. A driving aspect of international health informatics is that telecommunication technology, rehabilitative technology, intelligent home technology and many other components are moving together and form one integrated world of information and communication media. The complete series has been accepted in Medline. Volumes from 2005 onwards are available online.

Volume 148

Recently published in this series

Vol. 147. T. Solomonides, M. Hofmann-Apitius, M. Freudigmann, S.C. Semler, Y. Legré and M. Kratz (Eds.), Healthgrid Research, Innovation and Business Case – Proceedings of HealthGrid 2009

Vol. 146. K. Saranto et al. (Eds.), Connecting Health and Humans – Proceedings of NI2009 – The 10th International Congress on Nursing Informatics

Vol. 145. A. Gaggioli et al. (Eds.), Advanced Technologies in Rehabilitation – Empowering Cognitive, Physical, Social and Communicative Skills through Virtual Reality, Robots, Wearable Systems and Brain-Computer Interfaces

Vol. 144. B.K. Wiederhold and G. Riva (Eds.), Annual Review of Cybertherapy and Telemedicine 2009 – Advanced Technologies in the Behavioral Social and Neurosciences

Vol. 143. J.G. McDaniel (Ed.), Advances in Information Technology and Communication in Health

Vol. 142. J.D. Westwood, S.W. Westwood, R.S. Haluck, H.M. Hoffman, G.T. Mogel, R. Phillips, R.A. Robb and K.G. Vosburgh (Eds.), Medicine Meets Virtual Reality 17 – NextMed: Design for/the Well Being

Vol. 141. E. De Clercq et al. (Eds.), Collaborative Patient Centred eHealth – Proceedings of the HIT@HealthCare 2008 joint event: 25th MIC Congress, 3rd International Congress Sixi, Special ISV-NVKVV Event, 8th Belgian eHealth Symposium

Vol. 140. P.H. Dangerfield (Ed.), Research into Spinal Deformities 6

ISSN 0926-9630

Detection and Prevention of Adverse Drug Events

Information Technologies and Human Factors

Edited by

Régis Beuscart

Werner Hackl

and

Christian Nøhr

IOS Press

Amsterdam • Berlin • Tokyo • Washington, DC

ISBN 978-1-60750-043-8
Library of Congress Control Number: 2009932639

Publisher
IOS Press BV
Nieuwe Hemweg 6B
1013 BG Amsterdam
Netherlands
fax: +31 20 687 0019
e-mail: order@iospress.nl

Distributor in the UK and Ireland
Gazelle Books Services Ltd.
White Cross Mills
Hightown
Lancaster LA1 4XS
United Kingdom
fax: +44 1524 63232
e-mail: sales@gazellebooks.co.uk

Distributor in the USA and Canada
IOS Press, Inc.
4502 Rachael Manor Drive
Fairfax, VA 22032
USA
fax: +1 703 323 3668
e-mail: iosbooks@iospress.com

PRINTED IN THE NETHERLANDS

Detection and Prevention of Adverse Drug Events
R. Beuscart et al. (Eds.)
IOS Press, 2009

Preface

Along with the continuously increasing sophistication and refinement of diagnostic procedures and therapeutic processes, the risk of Adverse Events occurring during a patient's hospitalization is also steadily rising up.

Most of the modern medications have a powerful therapeutic impact balanced by equally threatening poisonous potential side effects. Thus the risk of Adverse Drug Events (ADE) is rocketing, partly due to medication errors.

That is why Quality of Care and Patient Safety have become a general concern shared by a large community of healthcare professionals and patients.

Different strategies have been tried for tracking ADEs: reporting systems have proven to be useful but they are not exhaustive; records and chart reviews are effective in the detection of ADEs and for an evaluation of their prevalence, but these methods are time-consuming and their reproducibility is questionable. Automatic detection of ADE is still in the research domain.

Nevertheless, at the bottom line, all the teams in the world are facing identical problems: how to reliably detect ADEs, how to efficiently prevent them. War stories about ADEs are all alike, whatever the country and whatever the setting: hemorrhage following an inattentive prescription of NSAID on a bleeding ulcer, renal insufficiency after heparin treatment, reactions to antibiotics and antiviral drugs, etc.

Properly managing the modern therapeutic drugs requires mastering a large quantity of information and a high level of complex knowledge, both probably exceeding human capacities. Therefore Information and Communication Technologies (ICT) are called in for additional help to access medical records, manage the data, enhance the knowledge, perform statistical analyses, and provide Decision Support.

But despite this powerful technology support many problems remain.

The characteristics of the Electronic Health Records (EHR) vary according to the suppliers, the hospitals, the countries. Coding systems can be different. Norms and standards vary from place to place. The extraction and exploitation of medical data from different sources then appear as a real challenge and cannot be solved without the definition of common data models, standard references, classifications and taxonomies.

The classification of drugs is in itself a tower of Babel: brand names, commercial names, ATC codes, various dosages, regimens, routes of administration, pharmacological effects, potential ADE or allergies, etc. The knowledge is mastered by a limited community of experts while the complexity of the interactions and the frequency of the side effects would require that this knowledge be shared by a large number of healthcare professionals and by the patients themselves.

Moreover, hospitals are much more than a mere technological setting: they are organized by administrative managers, they are ruled by physicians and nurses who are not robots, they treat citizens unwillingly playing the patient role. That is why organizational and human factors must be carefully studied as they can be at the origin or contribute to the occurrence of an ADE.

The new possibilities offered by statistical methods, data mining applications able to exploit large amount of records open a new era in the identification of abnormal hospitalization stays and detection of potential ADEs. Exploitation and screening of free-text documents such as letters and reports are now possible by means of semantic mining applications, providing new sources of patient information.

When looking at the papers gathered in this book, it appears that the approaches used to identify and prevent ADE are diverse but confronted to similar problems of codification, data exploitation, statistical analysis, etc. The ICT bring in powerful resources but they have to be driven by clear scientific objectives.

This workshop gathers knowledgeable and active persons in the domain, who are currently working at solving the problems. This is the opportunity to confront the ideas and the experiences stemming from various continents, and particularly from several EU projects financed to contribute to the resolution of the ADE problem. It is the occasion to find common ways for solving some of the difficulties everyone is sharing and make progress happen. Many thanks to Prof. David Bates, Prof. Johanna Westbrook for their participation and their keynotes; to Prof. Peter Elkin and Prof. André Kushniruk for their support and their clarifying interventions; to all the participants to the workshop; and to the European Commission which, by funding European Projects on this topics, allowed the organization of this workshop and the edition of this book.

Régis Beuscart, Werner Hackl and Christian Nøhr (Editors)
September 2009

Contents

Part A

Keynotes on Patient Safety

Detection and Prevention of Adverse Drug Events
R. Beuscart et al. (Eds.)
IOS Press, 2009

doi:10.3233/978-1-60750-043-8-3

Measuring Patient Safety: the Need for Prospective Detection of Adverse Events

David W. BATES, MD, MSc
Chief, Division of General Internal Medicine, Brigham and Women's Hospital
Medical Director of Clinical and Quality Analysis, Partners Healthcare
Director, Center for Patient Safety Research, Brigham and Women's Hospital
Board Chair, American Medical Informatics Association
And External Program Lead for Research, World Alliance for Patient Safety, WHO

While medical care is intended to improve health, all too often patients are harmed by the care they receive. A major reason that this issue was overlooked for so long is that institutions have relied on spontaneous reporting to detect injuries. However, spontaneous reporting detects only about one in twenty injuries caused by healthcare in hospitals. Thus, there is a clear need to develop approaches that allow organizations to measure in an on-going and prospective way the injuries that healthcare causes.

A growing body of research demonstrates that it is possible to do this, by using electronic tools to sift through clinical data and identify potential injuries, and then validate whether or not harm has actually occurred. This evidence will be reviewed for adverse events of all types, but there will be a specific focus on adverse drug events because of the focus of this workshop in this area. The strengths and limitations of approaches taken to date will be reviewed, including recent specific studies in this area. These demonstrate that it is possible at relatively low cost to identify adverse drug events even in institutions which do not have advanced information systems, by extracting pharmacy and laboratory data and looking for the presence of signals. These signals are then followed up, typically be a pharmacist.

At the conclusion of this talk, a set of challenges and next frontiers for work in this area will be discussed. It is likely that this work will become much easier with additional computerization of data, especially with increased use of electronic documentation.

Detection and Prevention of Adverse Drug Events
R. Beuscart et al. (Eds.)
IOS Press, 2009

doi:10.3233/978-1-60750-043-8-4

The Impact of Commercial Electronic Medication Management Systems on Errors and Clinicians' Work in Hospitals

Johanna I WESTBROOK[a]
[a] *Director, Health Informatics Research & Evaluation Unit, Faculty of Health Sciences, University of Sydney*

The intelligent use of electronic medication management systems is dependent upon a strong research foundation which investigates multiple indicators of system effectiveness and the mechanisms which drive both expected and unexpected outcomes. Two recent systematic reviews[1, 2] show the relatively scant evidence of the effectiveness of electronic prescribing systems to reduce prescribing errors. They demonstrate study limitations in terms of the generalisability of research findings, and the measurement complexities in assessing indicators of effectiveness. Changes in medication administration errors following electronic medication management system implementation have rarely been investigated and measurement of such changes also poses particular methodological challenges.

The integration and use of electronic medication management systems into health care organisations are influenced by information system, clinical, organisational and physical factors. The extent of integration will play a role in how systems are used and their overall impact on patient outcomes and organisational effectiveness and efficiency. Health care service delivery and information system implementation models are also drivers in determining the effects of systems on key performance indicators. Researchers are faced with the challenge of distinguishing what is possible to achieve from the ideal information system in the best-funded and organised health care organisation, to what is probable from an average information system implemented in a resource-constrained health care organisation. Thus a research agenda which focuses on measurement of context, mechanisms and outcomes[3] is appropriate.

In the last decade Australian health care organisations have increased investments in clinical information systems. As a predominantly public health care system, policy and decision-making have been guided by an emphasis on the procurement of commercial, integrated systems which have features generically applicable to a broad range of health care organisations. Business cases prepared by state and national governments to support large-scale investment in clinical information systems have relied heavily upon research evidence from overseas, predominantly the United States. However, acknowledging the roles that different health care delivery models, funding mechanisms, organisational and professional cultures may have on information system use and effectiveness, the need for local evidence of the effectiveness of systems in Australian health care organisations has become paramount to inform policy and implementation decision-making. Comparison of research conducted in different countries and settings facilitates a disentanglement of possible contextual and system factors which contribute to improvements in care delivery and outcomes.

This presentation describes a program of research[4] designed to develop innovative approaches to the measurement of the effectiveness of electronic medication management systems, and apply these systematically to establish an evidence-base to guide system design, implementation and use. The first component of the program has a focus on measuring the effectiveness of electronic medication management systems to reduce prescribing and medication administration errors and to promote safe medication practices. Results from controlled before and after studies of prescribing errors at multiple hospitals using different commercial medication management systems will be presented which examine overall changes in prescribing error rates, by type and severity. Observational methods and tools[5] applied to measure medication administration errors before and after system implementation will also be described. New types of medication errors, attributable to system use identified during these studies, will be illustrated.

The second component of the research program focuses on measuring how system use impacts on the work and communication practices of doctors and nurses. This is aimed at answering questions such as, whether use of electronic medication management systems 'saves' clinicians time, and whether this 'saved time' is devoted to direct care of patients. A work observation method by activity timing (WOMBAT)[6] will be discussed, including results of its application to quantify patterns of work and communication by hospital nurses and doctors.[7] A further element of this research which will be outlined is the application of video observational studies to identify how system use is integrated into clinical work flows, including how mobile technologies are used[8] and how physical space can influence where and how systems are used safely.

References

[1] Ammenwerth E, Schnell-Inderst P, Machan C, siebert U. The effect of electronic prescribing on medication errors and adverse drug events: A systematic review. J Am Med Inform Assoc. 2008;15(5):585-600.

[2] Reckmann M, Westbrook J, Koh Y, Lo C, RO D. Does computerized provider order entry reduce prescribing errors for hospital inpatients? A systematic review. J Am Med Inform Assoc. 2009;16(5):In press.

[3] Pawson R, Tilley N. Realistic Evaluation. London: Sage Publications Ltd; 1997.

[4] Westbrook J, Braithwaite J, Georgiou A, et al. Multi-method evaluation of information and communication technologies in health in the context of wicked problems and socio-technical theory. J Am Med Inform Ass. 2007;14(6):746-55.

[5] Westbrook J, Woods A. Development and testing of an observational method for detecting medication administration errors using information technology. Proceedings of 10th International Congress on Nursing Informatics. Amsterdam: IOS Press; 2009.

[6] Westbrook J, Ampt A. Design, application and testing of the Work Observation Method by Activity Timing (WOMBAT) to measure clinicians' patterns of work and communication. Int J Med Inform. 2009;78S(S25-S33).

[7] Westbrook JI, Ampt A, Kearney L, Rob MI. All in a day's work: an observational study to quantify how and with who doctors on hospital wards spend their time. Med J Aust. 2008;188(9):506-9.

[8] Andersen P, Lindgaard A, Prgomet M, Creswick N, Westbrook J. Is selection of hardware device related to clinical task?: A multi-method study of mobile and fixed computer use by doctors and nurses on hospital wards. Journal of Medical Internet Research. 2009;In press.

Detection and Prevention of Adverse Drug Events
R. Beuscart et al. (Eds.)
IOS Press, 2009

doi:10.3233/978-1-60750-043-8-6

Patient Safety Through Intelligent Procedures in Medication: The PSIP Project

Régis BEUSCART [a], Peter McNAIR [b], Jytte BRENDER [c] and the PSIP consortium
[a] *Lille University Hospital, Université de Lille –UDSL- EA2694, France*
[b] *Region Hovedstaden, Copenhagen, Denmark*
[c] *Aalborg University, Denmark*

Abstract. The European project Patient Safety through Intelligent Procedures in medication (PSIP) aims at preventing medical errors. The objective are: (1) to facilitate the systematic production of epidemiological knowledge on Adverse Drug Events (ADE) and (2) to improve the entire medication cycle in a hospital environment. The first sub-objective is to produce knowledge on ADE: to know, as exactly as possible, per hospital, per medical department, their number, type, consequences and causes, including human factors. Data Mining of structured hospital data bases, and semantic mining of free-texts will provide a list of observed ADE, with frequencies and probabilities, thus giving a better understanding of potential risks. The second sub-objective is to develop innovative knowledge based on the mining results and to deliver professionals and patients contextualized alerts and recommendations fitting the local risk parameters. This knowledge will be implemented in a PSIP-Platform independent of existing ICT applications.

Keywords. Patient Safety, Quality of Care, Adverse drug events, data mining, CPOE, CDSS.

Introduction

When a citizen enters a hospital to undergo exams or treatments, when he is given a doctor's prescription, delivered his medications by pharmacists or administered his drugs by a nurse, he expects it for the better of his health and welfare, he assumes that he will benefit from the medical service rendered. But the effectiveness of the therapies available nowadays should also be seen in perspective with the potentially negative consequences of the action ordered: Adverse Events. Consequently, each prescription exposes professionals and patients to have to handle risks both from a medical perspective (potential ADE) and from an economic perspective.

Adverse Events in healthcare and therefore patient safety have become a major public health issue. The health and economic indicators have been studied in all the industrialized countries in order to measure the extent of the phenomenon. Detailed figures are still difficult to obtain for Europe as a whole. But every national survey so far confirms the trends shown in US: in about 10% of the hospital admissions serious mistakes occur, and in about 60% of the cases medications are involved [1].

The incidence of ADE changes according to the age of patients. In France [2], they represent:

- 5 to 10% of the reasons for hospitalization of people over the age of 65
- 20% over 80 years
- 50% over 95 years.

With the expected ageing of the population, it is likewise that Adverse Drug reactions will become one of the main causes of mortality and morbidity in Europe, assuming that it is not one of them already, given the lack of exhaustive epidemiological data available regarding this phenomenon.

Most of the usually cited numbers are estimates and nationwide extrapolations issued from qualitative / quantitative regional studies. These studies are generally grounded on more or less large samples of healthcare records reviewed by experts [3,4]. Therefore, these numbers or estimates bear a relative uncertainty. Moreover, their methodological and statistical reliability can be questioned.

For the last twenty years, ICT applications have been developed and implemented in hospital settings. A huge amount of efforts have been made to incorporate in Electronic Health Record (EHR) or in Clinical Information Systems (CIS) specific applications to support the medication ordering, dispensing and administration functions. These applications are usually referred as Computerized Provider Order Entry (CPOE) systems.

As a consequence, a huge amount of data is available in EHR, Lab Management Systems and CPOE. More often, these data are only used for the management of the patients, or for medico-economic purposes. These data should also be utilized for a better knowledge on the population of hospitalized patients, a better comprehension of the hospitalization characteristics or modalities, and the assessment of the quality of care and epidemiologic studies.

Comparing, on one hand the difficulty to obtain reliable epidemiological information on ADE [4], on the other hand the availability of a large number of data recorded in the hospital information systems, is at the origin of the first objective of the PSIP Project: to identify, by innovative Data and Semantic Mining techniques, healthcare situations where patient safety is at risk. This implies to get a better knowledge of the prevalence of Adverse Drug Events and of their characteristics. This will be done by running semi-automatically data mining and semantic mining techniques on existing data repositories.

The second objective is to develop Decision Support Functions using the knowledge extracted by these methods. Indeed, a number of studies [5,6] have demonstrated that CPOE are efficient for improving productivity and quality of care and patient safety. In this respect, the most useful CPOE features involve some sort of Decision Support functions: patient specific dosing suggestions, reminders to monitor drug levels, reminders to choose an appropriate drug, checking for drug-drug interactions, standardized order sets, easy access to patient data and reference information while ordering.

So, the second objective consists in developing concepts and methods to improve the decision support tool related to the medication cycle, and deliver to healthcare professionals and patients usable, efficient and contextualized alerts and just-in-time point of care relevant information.

The main original concept in PSIP is CONTEXTUALIZATION. It is assumed that ADE occurrence is different according to the countries, the regions, the hospital, the medical department. To validate this hypothesis, data and semantic mining will be performed in those various situations, to record the frequency of potential or proven ADE. Consequently, rules based Clinical Decision Support System (CDSS) will have to be adaptable to those different concepts, particularly to avoid useless or over-alerting.

We will present here a global view of the project and of its achievements, particularly in the field of data mining and knowledge elicitation.

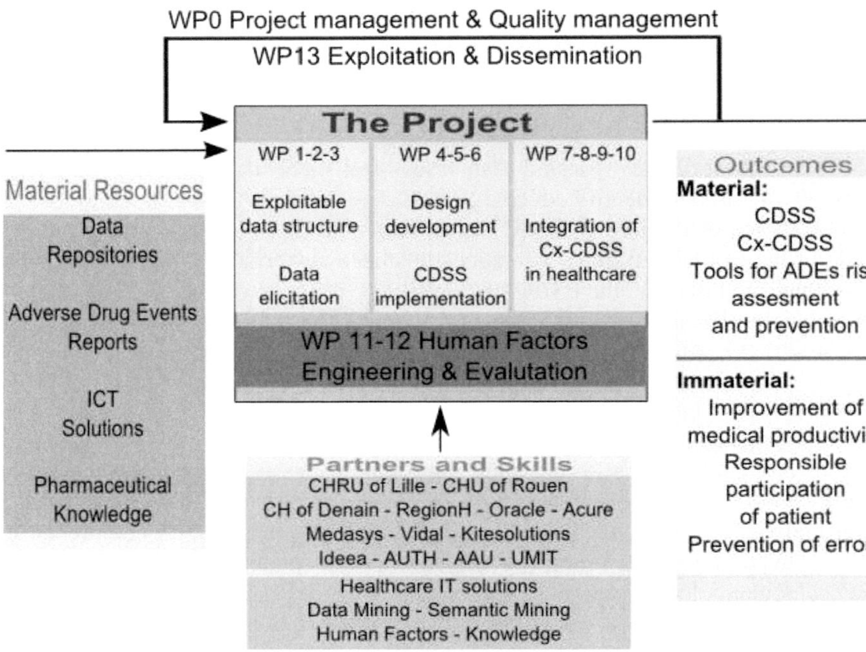

Figure.1. The global framework of the PSIP Project

1. Material and Methods

1.1. Datasets for Data and Semantic Mining

EHRs seem to be the best data source in the field of ADEs [2, 3]. A data model has been designed in the context of PSIP. It contains 8 tables and 92 fields and is used in a central repository.

This data model allows the extractions and exports of data under a common model. By this means, 2,600 hospitalization stays were extracted from RegionH hospitals (DK), including clinical, biological and CPOEs data. Similar 10,500 hospital records from the Denain General Hospital were extracted by means of scripts, in cooperation with the Medasys Company. 4,000 records are obtained from the Rouen University Hospital. 7,700 are currently extracted from the Lille Regional University Hospital.

All the medical data are anonymized and collected in a common repository. The management of this common repository includes an important verification phase and quality management. It is completely anonymous and no personal information can be retrieved.

The organization of such a common data repository makes necessary common coding of the clinical, biological, pharmaceutical data.

- Clinical diagnoses are coded using ICD10, which is in use in both Danish and French hospitals
- Lab results are coded using C-NPU (Committee on Nomenclature, Property and Units)
- Drugs are coded according to the ATC (Anatomical Therapeutic Chemical) classification system from the WHO Collaborating Center for Drug Statistics Methodology.

1.2. Data Mining Methods

To explore these large Hospital databases, statistical methods and data mining techniques are used to identify adverse events.

The choice of the most adapted Data Mining methods is not simple. A complete review of the available mining techniques has been performed to identify which were the most adapted to reach the PSIP objectives.

Two complementary steps are performed:

- Procedure A: to identify atypical groups amongst the patients; identify groups of patients that are potential ADE victims;
- Procedure B: for each effect (potential ADE), to establish the link between that effect and all the causes and contexts.

For Procedure A, the technique of Multiple Correspondence Analysis was employed.

For Procedure B, 3 techniques can be employed: Decision Trees, Association Rules, and Latent Classes analysis. This is supported by the fact that data mining techniques such as CART, Decision Trees, Association Rules, nearest neighbor techniques tend to be more robust when applied to "messy" real world data. Another reason is that the results of data mining techniques as CART or Decision Trees can provide knowledge that is easily transposable under the form of "rules" to be embedded in Clinical Decision Support Systems.

Using these complementary techniques allow for identifying medical cases that have a high probability to be ADE.

1.3. Semantic Mining Methods

Semantic Mining in the medical documents are techniques to extract relevant information from letters and reports: discharge letters, orders, procedure reports. Semantic Mining is performed using the F-MTI (a Multi-Terminology Extractor) Platform developed by the Rouen CISMEF Team [7]. The semantic mining of free text documents has proven to be efficient in the identification of drugs names and diagnoses.

A robot can then transform diagnoses in ICD10 codes and drug commercial or brand names in ATC codes.

This method has proven to be useful in two different situations.

1. In hospitals where no CPOE is installed, the semantic mining of the discharge letters give useful information on the drugs that have been prescribed and delivered during the hospitalization, as well as on the drugs prescribed at the discharge of the patient.

2. For all hospitals, the semantic mining of the discharge letter of the previous hospitalization can provide relevant information concerning the chronic diseases and the long term therapies of the patient. As more than 70% hospital stays concern chronic patients, the comprehension of the history and causes of the Adverse Event can be improved.

1.4. Validation of the Rules and Knowledge Elicitation

The validation of the knowledge obtained from data and semantic mining requires two types of methods: (1) validation of the rules and (2) validation of the clinical cases.
The rules associate information on drugs with lab results along with some clinical outcomes. For validation, these rules have to be confronted with the existing clinical and pharmacological knowledge available in the scientific literature or in specialized information repositories such as the VIDAL EXPERT System [8]. This process provides a scientific knowledge-based filtering and validation of the rules.

The abnormal stays identified by the data mining procedures are characterized by a large amount of data describing each patient's case. Only human experts such as specialized physicians may extensively review these data in order to decide whether the stay at hand presents or not a potential ADE. Complementary, this review allows assessing the capacity of the clinicians to understand the (sometimes complex) association rules, to assess the clinical relevance of the rules attached to the reviewed stay.

The review of the rules has allowed for validating more than 80 decision rules.

The review of the cases allowed a confrontation of the data mining results with the experts judgments. Realized by Human Factors experts, this review did not only provide a quantitative assessment of the system but also a qualitative evaluation on the potential role of PSIP for detecting and trying to prevent ADE in a daily practice.

1.5. Implementation and Design of Contextualized Clinical Decision Systems.

The process for knowledge model construction followed in PSIP is based on CommonKADS. This method is completely described in the paper from Vassilis Koutkias and coll. The implementation of the decision rules have been done using GASTON Software [9], which allows the representation of knowledge under various formats: primitives, problem-solving methods, and ontologies (domain ontologies and method ontologies).

The first implementation of the rules developed in PSIP has been done and proves the feasibility of the CDSS. Contextualization is currently done by means of different probabilities according to the frequency of ADE in different contexts.

2. Results

Only a brief summary of the results is presented in this section: each step is extensively described in other chapters of this book.

During the first year of the project, a data model has been proposed, validated and accepted. It has proven to be usable and useful, adapted to the following data mining phases. This data model is currently used in another European project.

Data and Semantic Mining have been experimented with good results. These mining techniques allow the selection of context-dependant knowledge rules as well as the identification of medical cases which can be potential ADEs.

In April 2009, 55 outcomes have been explored; generating 220 decision trees, from which 600 decision rules are automatically induces. After filtering and validation, 80 decision rules are fully validated and ready to be used and implemented in the CDSS. This process is under progress and continuously improved.

These rules are implemented through Gaston [9] and tested with real cases. This test has demonstrated that the CDSS is able to recognize the potential ADE cases in a data base of clinical records. Only 14 cases amongst more than 5,000 records were erroneous.

3. Discussion

In order to improve patient safety, quality of care and ultimately human performances, specific IT systems have been developed to support the medication ordering process. In hospital settings, most of these systems have been expanded to incorporate functions supporting the medication cycle, i.e. the prescribing phase performed by the physician, the administration phase usually performed by nurses and the dispensing phase achieved by the pharmacists. However, these features remain complex and might be available, efficient and usable in only a small number of well-known, well-studied home-grown situations. Commercial systems seem to be far less efficient and usable.

The PSIP Project aims at reinforcing and expanding existing technologies and making them more efficient, safe and acceptable. The semi-automatic identification of ADEs requires a precise evaluation. The DSS technology that has been envisaged requires Human Factors driven redesign, especially when considering their Human-Computer Interfaces (HCI) and mobile systems.

The first objective of the Project aims at identifying ADE cases in the hospital databases. The available data are obtained from clinical Electronic Health Record, Lab Management Systems, Reports, and CPOEs. By aggregating these data, and analyzing them with statistical tools, it is possible to identify cases where the common occurrence of certain clinical features, lab results and drug prescription make the probability of an ADE high.

Obviously, it is not proven that these cases were real ADE. Nevertheless, they are potential ADE; in many cases (more than 60%) the expert review confirmed the occurrence of an ADE.

Moreover the experts review is showing that the world is complex and not black/white. In many cases, contraindicated drugs were prescribed in presence of another drug or despite a diagnosis. But the experts reviewing the cases explained that in complex medical situations, involving multiple diseases, this medical attitude is comprehensible.

In conclusion, given the data at hand in hospital databases, the PSIP system is able to identify cases that have all the characteristics of a potential ADE.

The second objective of PSIP is to develop a platform incorporating CDSS modules to connect to healthcare IT applications, primarily CPOE, to deliver to healthcare professionals and patients usable, efficient and contextualized alerts and just-in-time and point of care relevant information. Since in existing decision support system the risk of over-alerting is high, many alerting systems are deactivated.

The PSIP Projects is more oriented toward the management of the risks associated to the prescription/administration of drugs in a complex or risky environment: how to manage drugs by laboratory or clinical monitoring; when and how to take into account the results of the monitoring; provide information in case of abnormalities in the monitoring or in case of absence of monitoring.

All these actions take place in medical units of hospital departments, with identified characteristics. The contextualization of the alerting/monitoring system is the chosen way for providing healthcare professionals with what can be the right information in the right place.

Human factors studies are indispensable to link the technical aspects of the project with the human and organizational dimensions. The continuous confrontation between medical, technical and HF experts within the project is one of the most efficient way of progress. It is expected that the Information Technology advances will meet the expectations of the healthcare professionals, improving patient safety, avoiding some ADE, without blaming anyone.

4. Conclusion

The PSIP project outcomes are both material and immaterial. Material outcomes come in the form of tools and methods for continuous Adverse Events risk management (assessment, detection, prevention) and for the continuous monitoring, updating and improvement of these tools. Material outcomes also include new contextualized knowledge-based modules, extended knowledge on healthcare situations at risk for patients, and identification of groups of patients likely to benefit from some sort of improvement in error prevention, in productivity and safety of the medical interventions, and an increased responsible participation of the patients in a position to take part on the control of their own therapeutic process.

Acknowledgement

The research leading to these results has received funding from the European Community's Seventh Framework Program (FP7/2007-2013), under Grant Agreement n° 216130 - the PSIP project.

References

[1] Sauer F, Patient & Medication Safety, EJHP-P 11 2005-4
[2] Appendix 36, French Health High Committee's 2004 report, available at http://www.securite-sociale.fr/hcaam/rapport2004/ann_hcaam_p2a.pdf
[3] Brennan TA, Gawande A, Thoma E, Studdert D. Accidental deaths, saved lives, and improved quality. N Engl J Med 2005 Sep 29;353(13):1405-9

[4] Murff HJ, Patel VL, Hripcsak G, Bates DW. Detecting adverse events for patient safety research: a review of current methodologies. J Biomed Inform. 2003 Feb-Apr;36(1-2):131-43.
[5] Garg A, Adhikari N, McDonald H, Rosas-Arenallo M, Devereaux P, Beyenne J, Sam J, Haynes R Effects of Computerized Clinical Decision Support Systems on Practitionner Performance and Patient Outcomes JAMA 2005, 293, 1223-1238
[6] Kawamoto K, Houlihan CA, Balas EA, Lobach DF. Improving clinical practice using clinical decision support systems: a systematic review of trials to identify features critical to success BMJ 2005: 330: 765
[7] Pereira S., Névéol A., Kerdelhué G., Serrot E., Joubert M., Darmoni S.J. Using multi-terminology indexing for the assignment of MeSH descriptors to health resources in a french online catalogue. AMIA Annu Symp Proc. 2008; 586-590.
[8] Vidal S.A. [cited 2009 April, 23]; Available from: http://www.vidal.fr/societe/vidal.
[9] de Clercq PA, Blom JA, Korsten HHM, Hasman A, Approaches for creating computer-interpretable guidelines that facilitate decisio support, Artif Intell Med (2004) 31(1), 1-27

Detection and Prevention of Adverse Drug Events
R. Beuscart et al. (Eds.)
IOS Press, 2009

doi:10.3233/978-1-60750-043-8-14

Human Factors Engineering for Computer-Supported Identification and Prevention of Adverse Drug Events

Marie-Catherine BEUSCART-ZÉPHIR [a, 1] and Christian NØHR [b]
[a] *Univ Lille Nord de France; INSERM CIC-IT-Evalab, Lille; CHU Lille; UDSL EA 2694; F-59000 Lille, France*
[b] *Department of Development and Planning, Aalborg University, Denmark*

Abstract. This paper addresses the question of the integration of Human Factors (HF) methods and models within projects aiming at (semi-) automatically identifying and preventing Adverse Drug Events (ADE). While more traditional methods such as voluntary reporting systems of medication errors tend to focus on HF causes of preventable ADEs, computer-based screening and mining methods tend to rely on a medical model of ADEs. As a consequence, HF methods and concepts are rarely considered in those projects. The paper describes the way HF methods have been incorporated in the PSIP (Patient Safety through Intelligent Procedures in medication) project lifecycle. It provides some examples of the results obtained and demonstrates their relevance to improve the entire detection and prevention process.

Keywords. Human Factors methods, ADE detection, ADE prevention, medication errors

Introduction

Drug ordering and administration is the most common therapeutic treatment for patients. Then not surprisingly, Adverse Drug Events (ADE) are the most common Adverse Events occurring during the care process [1]. This phenomenon is aggravated by the ever growing complexity of drugs, e.g. drug interactions and contra-indications, and ageing patient's multi-pathologies. These ADE result in human costs in terms of patients' deaths or injuries and economic costs in terms of hospital prolonged stays or lawsuits. Therefore, many countries consider ADE to be a major public health issue and currently invest a lot of resources in patient safety programs aiming at identifying, characterizing and preventing ADEs.

The European project PSIP (Patient Safety through Intelligent Procedures in medication) aims at contributing to this international effort of identification and prevention of ADE, by using innovative mining techniques of large medical databases coupled with contextualized Computer Supported Decision Systems (CDSS). In PSIP, human factors are considered a critical component of ADE characterization and prevention. Therefore Human Factors (HF) methods are closely intertwined with each

[1] Address for correspondence: Marie-Catherine Beuscart-Zéphir, Evalab, Faculté de Médecine, 1 Place de Verdun, 59000 Lille, France - mcbeuscart@univ-lille2.fr.

step of the project. This paper describes how the HF methods are integrated in the project and how they contribute to the research findings.

1. Background

1.1. Definition of ADE

Most of the researchers have adopted the Institute Of Medicine (IOM) definition of Adverse Event and Adverse Drug Event: "an injury due to medication management rather than the underlying condition of the patient" [1]. ADEs are usually divided into "preventable" and "non preventable". Preventable ADEs are assimilated to "medication errors" while non preventable ADEs are considered Adverse Drug Reactions that could not be avoided [2]. Medication errors are then defined as "the failure of a planned action to be completed as intended or the use of a wrong plan to achieve an aim" [1]. It is worth noting that not all the medication errors result in an ADE: most of them remain incidents or potential ADEs. Those strict definitions may pose some problems when considering the complexity of some therapeutic decision makings and the necessity for the healthcare professionals to balance the risk of the treatment, its expected benefit and the constraints linked with the physiological status of the patient. Physicians may be forced to prescribe drugs which they know are susceptible to provoke an ADE. The challenge is then to monitor the negative effect of the drug in order to maintain its impact within reasonable or acceptable range. In this approach, there is a continuum between the Non ADE / ADE situations, and there is also a continuum between preventable and non preventable ADEs and between Adverse Drug Events and Adverse Drug Reactions. There may also exist ADEs that are preventable but not considered as medical errors. In sum, an effort is necessary to refine the representation of ADE and to overcome the rigid definitions of ADE and preventable ADE. This clarification effort is not independent of the methods chosen to identify, characterize and prevent ADEs.

1.2. Systems for ADE Identification and Characterization

Different methods have been developed to identify and characterize ADEs and medication errors. Several classifications of these systems are available [3-5].They usually consider and combine the following dimensions:

- Active (voluntary reporting) vs. passive (involuntary reporting) systems
- Manual vs. automated
- Retrospective vs. prospective
- Focused on errors and incidents or on Adverse Drug Reactions (ADR, i.e. non preventable ADE)

Active systems or voluntary **reporting systems** of **medication errors or incidents** are the most ancient method, and it was imported in healthcare from other domains such as transportation (aviation) or Industry. Reporting systems are usually documented by healthcare professionals spontaneously or after prompting, but some systems are designed to be documented by the patients themselves. Those systems may be paper-based or electronically available[2]. Authors usually agree that all reporting systems suffer from important under-reporting biases. But as they contain narrative sections and tentative descriptions of the context and causative factors of the reported error or incident, they remain extremely useful for the analysis and characterization of contributing and mitigating factors of medication errors in healthcare, these factors being mainly of human and organizational nature. This knowledge is mandatory when it comes to the prevention and the design of counter-measures or safer work systems.

On site observation of the medication use process by trained observers belongs to passive systems and is equally useful to identify causative factors, especially human and organizational ones. This method is also interesting because it may prospectively identify dangerous situations. On site observations may be combined with other prospective analyses such as HFMEA (Healthcare Failure Mode and Effect Analysis). The major limitation of this method is again that it is very time consuming and somehow difficult to generalize.

The most important method in the passive systems category is the retrospective **Medical Chart Review**, which constitutes the main source of reliable epidemiological knowledge on ADE. At first these reviews were performed by trained experts, but despite its promising results, this method rapidly showed important limitations. Except when experts are intensively trained[4;6], the inter-experts agreement regarding the identification of ADE is usually moderate to low ($40 < k < 60$) [7] and even more so when experts are asked to validate the causative factors of the ADE ($k < .05$) [8]. Moreover the method is extremely time and resources consuming. As a consequence, researchers have tried to take the opportunity of the increasing availability of Electronic Health records to automate, at least partly, the reviewing process. The first systems relied on single data sources screening or mining, but they rapidly expanded to exploit integrated data sources (Hospital Information Systems - HIS, Electronic Medical Records - EMR, lab results, administrative data etc.). Except for a few systems targeting very specific Adverse Events in a circumscribed domain such as anaesthesia [9], to date no system has been able to reach complete automation, because of a too low specificity of the results. Therefore, manual experts review is still required on ADE identified automatically by those systems.

It is worth noting that those different categories of methods do not rely on the same models of ADE. Although most of the researchers adopt the IOM definition of ADE, the reality caught by reporting systems and on site observations on the one hand and medical chart reviews (whether paper or computer based) on the other hand is different.

Reporting systems of medication errors and incidents rely on an individual's perception and identification of an ADE. Even though the report is usually guided by a semi-structured reporting form, the medical data documented are limited to those selected by the reporting person. Most importantly, the report generally contains a narrative section and the description of probable causative factors, mostly of Human Factors nature. Given that human factors of all type are supposed to be the main contributing factor of medication errors [10] those reporting systems de facto rely on Human Factors based models of medication errors. This is clearly reflected in the existing taxonomies of ADE [11-13]. All those taxonomies have been elaborated from the analysis of existing reporting systems and databases of A(D)E in healthcare.

---

[2] There also exist national ADR reporting systems documented by healthcare professionals. These specific reporting systems do not target medication errors but rather yet unknown Adverse Drug Reactions. They contribute to pharmaco-vigilance systems.

On the contrary, Medical Charts Reviews / screening / mining rely on an extensive analysis of all available medical data, at least in the early stages of the review or screening. Semi-automated systems specifically search drug / lab results / diagnosis combinations to retrieve potential ADEs. But this investigation is limited to medical data: HF contributing factors are not recorded in the patient's file. As a consequence it may be considered that those systems rely mostly on a medical model of ADE.

1.3. Human Factors Contribution to ADE Identification and Prevention

Human Factors concepts and methods have long been contributing to patient safety studies and analyses [14]. Main contributions are (non exhaustive list):

- Support to the analysis of the healthcare work systems, in order to identify dangerous work situations, workarounds etc. [15]
- Models of individual and collective cognitive processes involved in medical decision making, models of human error, taxonomies of errors in the healthcare context [16]
- User-centered design of IT and CDSS systems for healthcare taking into account safety concerns for the patient; support to the analysis of healthcare professionals needs and requirements in terms of information management, decision making etc. [17]
- Usability evaluation and optimization of IT systems and medical devices [18]

But Human Factors methods have also been used to support the design and exploitation of the systems for identification of ADE:

- Reporting systems: support to the analysis of the reports, identification of contributing human and organizational factors
- Retrospective analyses of probable causes of errors and of contributing and mitigating factors such as Root Cause Analysis
- Prospective analysis in order to identify error prone situations (HFMEA)

As a consequence there exists a body of knowledge on **medication errors** in terms of contributing human factors of all types (organizational, cognitive, individual and collective). This knowledge is somehow incorporated in / expressed by existing taxonomies of medication errors or ADE [11-13].

It appears from the list above that human factor methods and concepts are used mostly in approaches to medication errors. Indeed, those methods and concepts are highly compatible with reporting systems of medication errors and incidents or with on site observation methods. But they are less compatible with Medical Chart Review methods and even less with automated identification systems of ADE, which do not capture the contributing and mitigating human factors of medication incidents or accidents. Indeed, to our knowledge, most of the projects aiming at developing automatic identification of ADE do not incorporate HF methods and concepts in their project lifecycle.

Nevertheless, the integration of HF issues in such projects is more than useful, it is mandatory. The ultimate goal of those projects is to change and improve the entire medication work system by delivering healthcare professionals ad hoc information in order to prevent the ADE to occur, in the form of Computer Decision Support System. Given the complexity of the medication prescribing – dispensing – administration cycle, any change to this work system should be sustained by concurrent HF analyses of the individual and collective work and cognitive processes and the CDSS design should be at least user-centered or even better user-driven. Such an approach would efficiently contribute limiting over-alerting and alert fatigue and would allow taking into account the collective dimension of the healthcare process by not limiting the CDSS functions to the prescribing physicians. Last but not least, the integration of the HF methods and concepts helps anticipating and balancing the benefits of the new CDSS functions with their potential negative effects on the overall work system (unexpected or unintended negative effects of Healthcare IT systems).

The following sections describe the HF methods that have been integrated in the PSIP project and provide illustrations of the findings and contributions to the project results.

2. Methods

Projects aiming at (semi-) automatically identifying and preventing ADEs follow a number of mandatory successive steps that structure the projects' lifecycles. A typical project lifecycle is depicted in the left column of Figure 1.

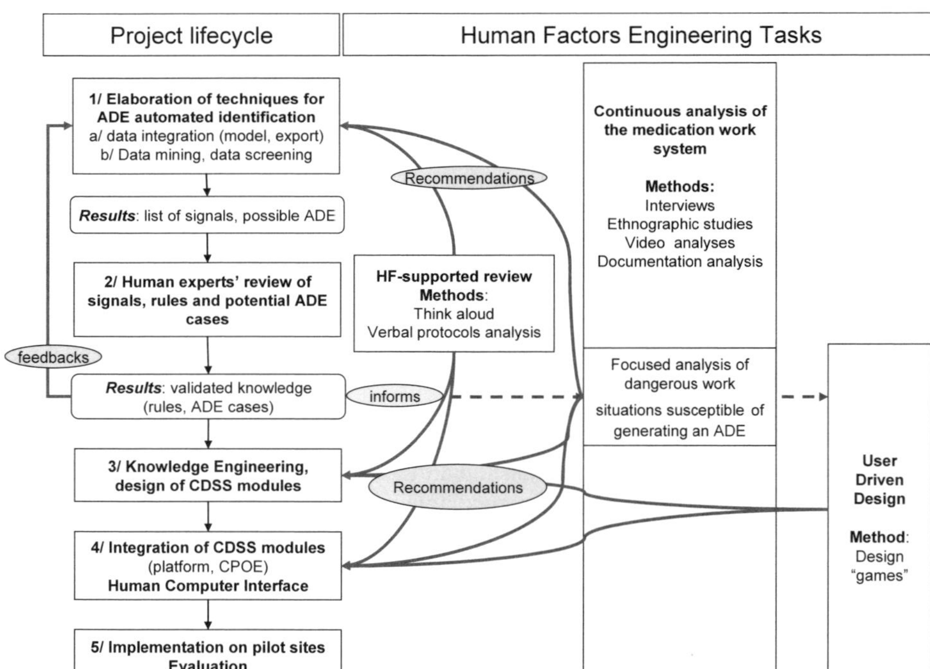

Figure 1. Overview of the integration of HF engineering tasks with the project lifecycle. The project lifecycle is depicted in the left column of the figure. Plain arrows indicate feedbacks or recommendations issued from HF results to the main steps of the system design. The dotted arrow shows how the results of the project inform the corresponding HF tasks.

Step 1 is the elaboration of the techniques for identification of possible ADE cases. It consists in collecting / exporting / integrating relevant data from different sources (HIS, Computerized Provider Order Entry – CPOE systems, Lab systems etc.), and then in screening or mining these data to identify abnormal cases susceptible of showing an ADE. Step 2 consists in the review and validation by human experts of the list of possible ADE cases and rules generated at step 1. When ADE cases are automatically identified, it is mandatory that human experts review, filter and validate /invalidate a representative sample of Normal / Abnormal cases to assess the validity of the system. This second step issues a validated knowledge to be used by step 3 and implemented in a CDSS system. Step 4 aims at integrating the CDSS modules into existing applications (CPOE, pharmacy systems) or at designing an independent platform and its corresponding Human Computer Interface allowing healthcare professionals to access this knowledge. Finally step 5 would consist in implementing the system in pilot sites and evaluating its performance in terms of diminution of ADEs.

In PSIP, different HF methods are used at the different steps of the project.

- All along the project lifecycle, an analysis of the medication use process work systems is performed. This analysis may rely on standard HF methods such interviews and ethnographic studies [19], or on more innovative ones such as video analyses [20]
- The mandatory experts' review of the data and semantic mining results is combined in PSIP with specific HF methods such as Think Aloud and use of portable usability labs in order to analyze the experts reasoning on possible ADE cases [21]
- The design phase of the CDSS modules and of their HCI is supported by innovative user driven methods [22]

All those methods may provide feedbacks and recommendations for all the stages of the PSIP project:

- Refinement of the data model and data mining techniques
- Design and contextualization of the CDSS modules
- Integration in existing applications and /or design of a specific platform's HCI

3. Results

The purpose of this paper is not to describe in detail the results obtained with each method and at each step of the project but rather to provide an overview of the type of contribution issued by the set of HF tasks. All the HF tasks are running in parallel, and for most of them preliminary results are available [19;21;22]. Table 1 displays a sample of interesting results obtained with each HF method and providing significant feedbacks or recommendations for each step of the project. For example, an important result of the interviews and on site observations is the identification of the prominent role of the nurse in all the steps of the medication use process, including the ordering one. The corresponding recommendation, addressed to the PSIP partners in charge of the design of the CDSS modules, is to identify the nurse role as an interesting candidate for the delivery of CDSS information. Similarly, the analysis of experts' verbalizations during the reviewing process allows identifying missing information such as blood sugar or blood pressure. The corresponding recommendation is addressed to the PSIP partners in charge of data model, data exports and data mining.

Table 1. Examples of results obtained with the various HF methods integrated in the PSIP project. For each result the possible corresponding recommendation for the refinement of the mining techniques or for the design of the CDS system are displayed

Continuous analysis of the work situation in the medication use process: Prescribing/ordering - dispensing – administration		
Method used	**Example of result**	**Corresponding recommendation**
Interviews and on site observations	In many organizations, the nurse is actively involved in the prescribing stage; she provides useful information and reminders to the physician. For most of the biochemical orders, she is also in charge of collecting the samples (urine, blood), sending them to the lab and of retrieving the lab results.	Most of the PSIP knowledge comes in the form of a combination of lab results and drug information. The information provided by the CDS System should not be limited to the prescribing physician, but also delivered to the nurse, possibly depending on which shift the nurse is on.
Model of the physician's decision making when ordering a drug	The decision making for drug ordering is composed of successive steps: information gathering, information interpretation, decision making, orders documentation.	When an alert is sent after the orders have been documented in the system, it is disruptive for the cognitive process. The physician has to retrace the entire process and start again with the information gathering phase. As far as possible, the relevant information should be delivered early on, during the information gathering phase
Observation of work practice in prescription of drugs	Decisions are made very distributed in time and localization, and usually prior to opening the CPOE system. The CPOE system is used as a data entry tool.	Design of decision support should not focus on alerts in the CPOE system alone. Alerts and advice should happen when and where decisions are made in order not to disrupt the cognitive process.
Observation of dispensing and administration of drugs	The work practice in dispensing and administrations is different according to experience and busyness among the nurses	Decision support for dispensing and administration is of a fundamental different character, and experiments are needed to develop an appropriate design approach.

Experts' review of the automatically identified ADE cases and corresponding rules		
Method used	**Example of result**	**Corresponding recommendation**
Analysis of experts' behavior (navigation)	The experts always start the review of a case by reading the discharge letter (or any other available document). They retrieve information not available in the database such as the patient's personal (home) treatment and clinical diagnoses.	The semantic mining could efficiently supplement the data mining by retrieving the patient's home treatment which is often cited in the transfer or discharge letter but rarely documented in the CPOE
Analysis of experts' behavior	The experts are interested in concomitant variations of drugs and lab results. Some of them try to display both in the same window. They appreciate lab results displayed as curves	The information displayed by the CDSS should aim at juxtapose drug information and related lab results. The system should offer the possibility of configuring the lab results display either as numbers (tables) or as curves
Analysis of verbal protocols	The experts miss some information such as blood sugar and blood pressure. These items are usually retrieved and documented by the nurse in the nurse record and not documented in the medical record.	Improve the data export (and extend the data model) to retrieve significant information documented only in the nurse records

Analysis of verbal protocols	The experts may agree with the PSIP association rule, agree there is an ADE, but they contest the relevance of the rule for the case at hand. The most frequent reasons are alcoholic patients, patients undergoing chemotherapy or patients in final state of illness (dying patients).	The CDS system could improve the contextualization of the PSIP modules by weighing the rules according to some typical diseases such as alcoholism and cancers treated by chemotherapy.

Design of the CDSS system and of its HCI		
Method used	**Example of result**	**Corresponding recommendation**
Design game to produce functional specifications.	Conceptual machine that can help to prevent the adverse event in the scenario presented in the design game..	Pop-up alerts are discarded. Integration and simultaneous presentation of essential information preferably in graphics.
Iterative prototyping	First draft paper mock-up presented to users and iteratively developed into a prototype tested in a simulation laboratory.	The decision support demanded by the clinicians is a mixture of smart presentation of information, guideline advice on additional tests and suggestions of alternative drugs

4. Discussion

From this short overview of the results it appears that the integration of Human Factors Engineering tasks within the project lifecycle provides useful feedbacks at all steps of this project.

The qualitative analysis of experts' comments and thinking while reviewing the suspected ADE cases produces valuable information for enriching the data model and for better tuning the data mining and semantic mining procedures, therefore efficiently supporting successive iterations and improvements of the ADE detection part of the PSIP system. Moreover, this qualitative approach has allowed identifying the main elements and dimensions both Danish and French experts rely on to make their decision. Consequently, the questionnaire supporting the computer supported review of the cases has been modified and extended to systematize the experts rating on those dimensions. This will allow freeing the future iterations of the reviewing from the think aloud method, which is more demanding on the experts and highly time consuming for the analysis of the results. This extended questionnaire could be generalized to other projects aiming at (semi-) automatically identifying ADE.

Field studies focused on the analysis of the medication use system, cognitive models of the users' cognitive processes and user driven innovation methods provide critical information to support the design of the CDSS system. It is well known that CDSS for healthcare professionals are a big usability and acceptance challenge [23;24]. Most of the CDSS come in the form of alerts that are disruptive of the cognitive processes, inadequate in the clinical context, and frequently overridden by exasperated or careless physicians. In most of other projects aiming at automating the detection and prevention of ADE, the lack of consideration of HF issues results in systems targeting mainly the prescribing physician at the ordering stage of the medication use process, and eventually the pharmacist at the control stage of the medication orders. The field studies carried out in the context of the PSIP project corroborate previous results of HF studies of the medication use process [25]. This work system is a highly complex and collaborative one, characterized by a distributive cognition organization. For the time being, and at least in the two cultures under observation (French and Danish hospitals), the nurse appears to be frequently involved in the ordering stage, to have the essential role in (dispensing) preparing and administering the meds, and to be in charge of managing the lab results. Therefore, the PSIP CDSS should also target this key user, possibly with an adapted format and display of information.

Finally, the major problem that still has to be intensively worked on is the clarification of the definition of the ADE targeted by automated systems. Other similar projects [6] may try to force compliance with the "standard" definition of ADE, for example by training their reviewing experts intensively on the Naranjo scoring. This procedure allows them to reach extremely high levels of inter experts agreement for both ADE identification and rating of causative factors ($k > .88$). However, the results obtained in the PSIP project from all categories of HF studies may question this option. The strict definitions of ADE, preventable ADE and medication errors are not compatible with the kind of "Events" identified in PSIP. Indeed, a part of these events may be considered "errors" therefore justifying the standard "alerting" model. But a significant part of the events identified tackle the risk part inherent to any therapeutic decision making. Supporting the collective monitoring and management of this risk appears to be the real challenge faced by the future PSIP CDS system.

5. Conclusion

This paper has presented an overview of the integration of the Human Factors Engineering tasks in the PSIP project lifecycle. It has illustrated the benefit of this approach for projects aiming at automatically identifying ADE and at delivering the healthcare professionals ad hoc information to prevent the ADE to occur. The history of ADE identification and prevention shows that those systems are currently the most promising and efficient ones [3;6;26]. Progressively shifting from voluntary reporting of medication errors methods to automated systems of ADE detection has implicitly made the conception of "Adverse Drug events" evolve. Clarifying this essential concept remains the most important challenge for the current projects. The Human Factors Engineering approach may help addressing this critical issue.

Acknowledgement

The research leading to these results has received funding from the European Community's Seventh Framework Programme (FP7/2007-2013) under grant agreement n° 216130 – the PSIP project.

References

[1] Institute Of Medicine, Preventing Medication Errors. The National Academic Press, Washington, DC, 2007.

[2] Murff HJ, Patel VL, Hripcsak G, and Bates DW, Detecting adverse events for patient safety research: a review of current methodologies. J.Biomed.Inform 36: 131-143, 2003.

[3] Bates DW, Evans RS, Murff H, Stetson PD, Pizziferri L, and Hripcsak G, Detecting Adverse Drug Events using Information Technology. The Journal of the American Medical Informatics Association 10: 115-128, 2003.

[4] Morimoto T, Gandhi TK, Seger AC, Hsieh TC, and Bates DW, Adverse drug events and medication errors: detection and classification methods. Qual Saf Health Care 13: 306-314, 2004.

[5] Amalberti R, Gremion C., Auroy Y., Michel P., Salmi R., Parneix P., Quenon J. L., and Hubert B. Typologie et méthode d'évaluation des systèmes de signalement des accidents médicaux et des évènements indésirables. 2006.

[6] Kilbridge PM, Campbell UC, Cozart HB, and Mojarrad MG, Automated surveillance for adverse drug events at a community hospital and an academic medical center. J.Am.Med.Inform Assoc. 13: 372-377, 2006.

[7] Thomas EJ, Lipsitz SR, Studdert DM, and Brennan TA, The reliability of medical record review for estimating adverse event rates. Ann.Intern.Med. 136: 812-816, 2002.

[8] Arimone Y, Miremont-Salame G, Haramburu F, Molimard M, Moore N, Fourrier-Reglat A, and Begaud B, Inter-expert agreement of seven criteria in causality assessment of adverse drug reactions. Br.J.Clin.Pharmacol. 64: 482-488, 2007.

[9] Benson M, Junger A, Michel A, Sciuk G, Quinzio L, Marquardt K, and Hempelmann G, Comparison of manual and automated documentation of adverse events with an Anesthesia Information Management System (AIMS). Stud Health Technol Inform 77: 925-929, 2000.

[10] Schmidt E, Le risque médicamenteux nosocomial. Circuit hospitalier du médicament et qualité des soins. Masson, Paris, 1999.

[11] World Health Organization. The Conceptual Framework for the International Classification for Patient Safety. 2009. 24-5-2009.

[12] Chang A, Schyve PM, Croteau RJ, O'Leary DS, and Loeb JM, The JCAHO patient safety event taxonomy: a standardized terminology and classification schema for near misses and adverse events. Int.J.Qual Health Care 17: 95-105, 2005.

[13] National Coordinating Council for Medication Error Reporting and Prevention. NCC MERP: The First Ten Years"Defining the Problem and Developing Solutions". 2005. 23-5-2009.

[14] Carayon P, Human Factors and Ergonomics in Health Care and Patient Safety. In: Handbook of Human Factors and Ergonomics in Health Care and Patient Safety,(Ed. Carayon P), pp. 3-21. Lawrence Erlbaum Associates, New Jersey: 2007.

[15] Koppel R, Wetterneck T, Telles JL, and Karsh BT, Workarounds to barcode medication administration systems: their occurrences, causes, and threats to patient safety. J.Am.Med.Inform.Assoc. 15: 408-423, 2008.

[16] Zhang J, Patel VL, Johnson TR, and Shortliffe EH, A cognitive taxonomy of medical errors. J.Biomed.Inform. 37: 193-204, 2004.

[17] Malhotra S, Laxmisan A, Keselman A, Zhang J, and Patel VL, Designing the design phase of critical care devices: a cognitive approach. Journal of Biomedical Informatics 38: 34-50, 2005.

[18] Beuscart-Zephir MC, Elkin P, Pelayo S, and Beuscart R, The human factors engineering approach to biomedical informatics projects: state of the art, results, benefits and challenges. Yearb.Med.Inform. 109-127, 2007.

[19] Riccioli C, Leroy N, and Pelayo S, The PSIP approach to account for Human Factors in Adverse Drug Events: preliminary field studies. In: Patient Safety through Intelligent Procedure in medication (Ed. Beuscart R.). IOS Press, 2009.

[20] Nøhr C and Botin L, Methodolgy for analysis of work practice with video observation. In: 3rd International Conference on Information Technology in Health Care: Socio-technical approaches (Eds. Westbrook JI, Coiera E, Callen J.L., and Aarts J), pp. 291-297. IOS Press, 2007.

[21] Leroy N, Luyckx M, Lecocq P, Marcilly R, and Beuscart-Zephir MC, Contribution of Human Factors for the review of automatically detected ADE. In: Patient Safety through Intelligent Procedure in medication (Ed. Beuscart R.). IOS Press, 2009.

[22] Kanstrup AM and NØHR C, Gaming against Medical Errors: methods and results from a design game on CPOE. In: Patient Safety through Intelligent Procedure in medication (Ed. Beuscart R.), 2009.

[23] Kuperman GJ, Bobb A, Payne TH, Avery AJ, Gandhi TK, Burns G, Classen DC, and Bates DW, Medication-related clinical decision support in computerized provider order entry systems: a review. J.Am.Med.Inform.Assoc. 14: 29-40, 2007.

[24] van der SH, Aarts J, van GT, Berg M, and Vulto A, Turning off frequently overridden drug alerts: limited opportunities for doing it safely. J.Am.Med.Inform Assoc. 15: 439-448, 2008.
[25] Beuscart-Zephir MC, Pelayo S, Anceaux F, Maxwell D, and Guerlinger S, Cognitive analysis of physicians and nurses cooperation in the medication ordering and administration process. Int.J.Med.Inform., 2006.
[26] Bates DW, O'Neil AC, Boyle D, Teich J, Chertow GM, Komaroff AL, and Brennan TA, Potential identifiability and preventability of adverse events using information systems. J.Am.Med.Inform.Assoc. 1: 404-411, 1994.

Detection and Prevention of Adverse Drug Events
R. Beuscart et al. (Eds.)
IOS Press, 2009

doi:10.3233/978-1-60750-043-8-25

Decision Support to Avoid Medication Errors - How Far Have We Come in Denmark and What Are the Present Challenges

Annemarie HELLEBEK [a, 1] and Christianna MARINAKIS [a]
[a] *The Copenhagen Unit for Patient Safety, Danish Society for Patient Safety and Infomatum A/S*

Abstract. The number of medication errors reported to The Danish National Board of Health in Denmark exceeds 5000 per year. It is well known that computerized physician order entry (CPOE) with addition of decision support tools may reduce the frequency of medication errors. The primary scope of the work in Denmark has been to help health care professionals avoiding harmful errors. Using data primarily from The Danish National Board of Health, based on the reports of errors from Danish hospitals,,and with our previous foundation in the international literature, we analyzed the errors which led to harmful conditions or death. In the process we developed a methodical consensus for identifying which medicines should have a warning attached, and we systematized the different kind of warnings. The following validation of the data resulted in a final list of 14 classes of drugs or drug substances, which all have been involved in serious medication errors. At present time there is a total of 136 different medicines with warnings found in the drug database for health professionals from Infomatum A/S (www.medicin.dk). In a parallel matter other decision support tools from Infomatum A/S[2] are available or in progress e.g. ensuring use of correct dosage based on normal range, information about drugs used during pregnancy.etc. A major challenge when implementing decision support for medication processes has been to ensure useful coding of the medicines, as there does not exist one unique identification number for each drug substance.

Introduction

The medication process in a hospital is a highly complex process involving a high number of choices from different health care professionals. First the correct medicine must be ordered for the disease and the choice must be modulated to accustom other treatments or specific conditions in the patient. Secondly the doctor must document the medicine for the pharmacist or nurse to dispense at the right time in the correct dose. When the medicine is dispensed it must be administered to the right patient using the right route – and if the administration route is by injection the velocity must be correct. After the administration the patient must be observed for effect and possibly side effects of the medicine. More than 5000 medication errors were reported in the Danish reporting system for adverse events in 2008. The reporting is anonymous but

[1] Corresponding Author: annemarie.hellebek@hvh.regionh.dk
[2] Infomatum A/S is a company jointly owned by The Danish Drug Information and The Danish Medical Association. Infomatum A/S publishes drug information for health professionals and the public.

compulsory among health professionals in hospitals, and soon (in 2010) it will expand to include primary care as well. The pattern of errors have been thoroughly reviewed twice (1,2) by the National Board of Health. The reviews suggest that the severity of the errors for the patient is related to both the drug step in the medication process and the type of error i.e. whether the error concerns picking out the wrong patient or the wrong dose or the wrong medicine. Medicines result in harmful errors in approximately 1% of the error reports. Some medicines are more frequently involved in harmful errors than others. These medicines are called high alert medicines or high risk medicines (3). In Denmark the primary focus on decision support has been to create systems for the health professionals in order to avoid harm from high risk medicines, secondly to reduce frequent types of less harmful events. Every time a health professional reports a medication error in a Danish hospital, the report is sent to one of the 5 regions, in which the hospital is situated. Subsequently the report is sent to The Danish National Board of Health,. In Infomatum A/S we identify which medicines have result in the most serious and harmful incidences (the SAC-3 cases). These medicines get a warning attached, which users of www.medicin.dk can see, when they look up the drug description on-line (free access). A major challenge for Infomatum A/S in developing decision support is, that no unique identification number exist for each active drug substance. This means, that every time a relevant active drug substance that should have patient safety warnings is picked all other drugs with the same active drug substance and dosage forms on the Danish market have to be manually identified, as they all should have the same warnings.. To achieve this is an international challenge, which if solved, could make a huge contribution to the way medical data id systemized worldwide.

1. Analysis of Decision Support Tools for the Medication Process

1.1. Methods

Presently most Danish hospitals and all Danish primary care physicians use CPOE for prescribing medicines. Specific knowledge on drugs can in some clinical situations be of crucial importance, a fact that led Infomatum A/S to develop a system of active and passive decision support. This feasibility is based on an existing and advanced database with detailed information on all registered medicines in Denmark (www.medicin.dk and printed versions). All drug information may be connected and integrated with the ordering systems in any desirable way.

In order to investigate the possibility of adding decision support into the drug information system The Danish Society for Patient Safety and Infomatum A/S under took a large literature review in 2004 (4).

1.2. Results

The review indicated that

- decision support systems must be easily accessible
- the rules in the systems should be accepted by the professionals
- if there should be warnings these should result from serious and preventable situations, and not be too many to avoid alarm fatigue.

A short version of the review underwent peer review and was published in the Danish Medical Journal in order to create discussion among professionals (5).

The study led to the conclusion, that decision support tools were desirable, and Infomatum A/S undertook the challenge developing them.

2. High Risk Drugs

After the analysis of the literature on decision support and the results of the first analysis of medication errors from The Danish National Board of Health, it was decided by Infomatum A/S, that an attempt should be made to develop warnings for medicines used in Denmark, which have caused hospitalization, handicap or death (SAC-3 events). The project was supported by a large foundation. It is worthwhile mentioning the importance of the Danish compulsory system of reporting errors. Without it, the project of high risk drugs would be of more theoretical use, and would not have developed to such a concrete set of warnings, as the case is today.

2.1. Methods

First 811 order errors reported between 2002 and 2004 were studied to elucidate further which medicines were high risk drugs in medicine ordering. 18 of the errors resulted in severe harm or death.

Secondly all medication errors between 2004-2006 published in the report from The Danish National Board of Health (2) and cases from the Danish Medical Complaint System (www.pkn.dk) were reviewed. 26 serious errors in the medication process were registered in the report from The Danish National Board of Health; 50% of these errors where caused by antihyperglycaemic agents, opioids, cardiovascular drugs or methotrexate. Review of cases from the complaint system did not add new medicines.

Third The Danish Medical Journal was reviewed for short notices on complications caused by severe medication errors in hospitals, and international literature on the subject was studied.

2.2. Results

The study group gained information on the causes of severe medication errors reported in Denmark over the years 2002-2006. The information was used to create a list of 136 medicines – either classes of drugs or specific drug substances. The list contained almost the same medicines as similar lists from abroad (see following list) (6).

List of classes of drugs or drug substances involved in serious medication errors in Denmark from 2002-2006 with warnings in www.medicin.dk:

- Acetylcystein
- Adrenaline
- Amiodarone
- Digoxin
- Phosphenytoin

- Gentamicin
- Insulin
- Potassium
- Methotrexate
- Opioidagonists
- Nevirapin
- NSAID
- Thiopental
- Warfarin

The study group invited a group of 18 hospital risk managers in order to discuss the list with local staff, and requested their return of comments. A similar invitation was sent to a steering committee for the study.

The process resulted in deletion of penicillin (risk of allergy) and paracetamol (risk of overdose) from the list. Penicillin was removed due to practitioners' fear of alarm fatigue, while paracetamol was removed due to the incomplete case report available. In spite of the seriousness of the described situation, it was unlikely, that paracetamol was the cause of the patient´s death.

Some risk managers mentioned that the warnings should appear only in connection to the relevant dosage form of the medicine and not necessarily in all medicines where the active drug substance is present, i.e. some warnings for morphine are only relevant for the injections - not for the patch.

In addition the list was also shown to the board of the Danish Society for Patient Safety constituting all important stakeholders. They argued that a large group of medicines for mild pain or arthritis "NSAID´s" should be added because of risk of gastric ulcer. This adverse drug event is quite frequent – but not always associated with serious damage or death. Although the study group initially had not included this class of drugs, they were soon added, as they fulfil the inclusion criteria of factual harm because of their frequent use in hospital settings.

The list is now published as a passive decision support tool in www.medicin.dk (7). Within the next year we hope some of the Danish regions will implement the tool all the way into their CPOE. In that way the information can become active in the sense,that each hospital can choose for itself, how and when they want the warnings, and what procedures to follow, when the warnings appear on the screen during prescription or administration of the drug.

3. Decision support in pregnancy and avoidance of wrong doses

Infomatum A/S has developed other decision support tools in the field of toxicology and patient safety. All medicines are provided with the latest evidence based information on their safety during pregnancy or nursing (breast feeding). The aim of this information is to give clinicians reliable guidelines on drug of choice, when prescribing un-avoidable medication for pregnant women e.g. antibiotics. In addition to this tool Infomatum A/S is at the time being working on maximum doses (as recommended by Micromedex and medical literature) for most active substances in the database. This will prepare the systems for warnings if the normal doses - based on clinical experience - are exceeded. This tool could create some problems, because hospital doctors sometimes want to exceed a recommended normal dose – and at other times, for instance in case of renal insufficiency, a normal dose may be far too high. This tool therefore has to be incorporated in patient specific data i.e. weight to become really useful. We have two challenges in this field.

In Denmark most notes in the patient chart are not yet electronic – the addition of weight etc. has to be performed manually. The other challenge is that we have to establish consensus among clinicians on algorithms for the correct dosage in renal insufficiency.

4. Decision Support to Avoid Interactions

Another tool for the medication order process is on-line help to avoid harmful interactions between the medicines. Traditionally the golden standard decision support tool for this control has been a book, “Hanstens”, which is updated every three months and known only to clinical pharmacologists. The ordinary clinical doctor would use Infomatum A/S´s database, accessible to the public as medicin.dk (either on one of the electronic platforms available, or as the printed versions). Medicin.dk includes primarily potential interactions identified by the companies at marketing and actual interactions identified after marketing. A few years ago it was decided, that a national interaction database (www.interaktionsdatabasen.dk) should be created to make it easy for professionals to identify interactions. To give the content as much scientific validity as possible, it was agreed that only interactions mentioned in the peer reviewed literature should be included. The database is now run by the Danish Medicines Agency reviewing the literature and adding information to the database.

But unfortunately we have ended up with two systems – medicin.dk using one data source and the national interaction database using another. Althought all serious interactions (marked with red in the national interaction database) are included in medicin.dk it is a present challenge to make these ends meet – for practitioners to look up interactions only in one place.

5. Decision Support Embedded in CPOE and Identification of Medicines

Decision support embedded in CPOE typically include allergy warnings, warnings against double ordering of the same drug and warnings against dispensing the wrong drug (using barcodes). The rules behind these tools require (only) unique identification of the drugs and for allergy warnings also information about the patient´s allergy status.

The ATC code system has been an effective way of systematize drug information in books. The use of the ATC code system in electronic prescribing and decision support created unforeseen problems in allergy detection/allergy warning systems, because some medicines (about 50) had more than one ATC code due to several indications and combination - drugs. Thus when a doctor codes for allergy for a drug with a specific ATC code- he or she might not be aware, that the same active substance could appear in another drug with no warning because it had another ATC code as well.

Other systems base their drug information on the generic names. Generic names work well except that one active substance may be registered under several generic names for different indications.

Finally neither the generic names nor the ATC codes differentiate between different forms of the medicine (tablets, injection etc.).

In Denmark we luckily have the Drug Medication Identifier (DrugID), which is a unique number. Every single drug can have many DrugID´s, one for every dosage and strength of the drug. This unambiguous coding enables Infomatum A/S to offer specific and tailored information in all imaginable combinations, whatever it is on high risk medicines, maximum dosage or allergy warnings. A remaining challenge exists: an active drug substance e.x methotrexate as tablets 2.5 mg has at the same time five different DrugID´s, one for each medical company making this drug at this strength and dosage form, which all have to be taken into account when coding.

6. Discussion

Rules for warnings against wrong use of high risk medicines could be established through a consensus process in Denmark. Development of the warnings were a major challenge e.g. choosing the right method of selecting the information, inclusive criteria for the warnings, the clinical evaluation and relevance etc. Here the co-operation with enthusiastic clinicians is of crucial importance not to mention the need for the reporting of errors as well. The warnings have so far been released as a passive decision support tool by Infomatum A/S in the on-line and public accessible Danish drug information system (www.medicin.dk).

A warning system for interactions released previously has not yet been successful due to lack of completeness in warnings. Other decision support tools like recommandations during pregnancy from Infomatum A/S have been a succes, but also challenging as the information may not always be consistent with the official warnings from the medical companies.

All decision support tools need a properly coded formulary. This requires modulation of existing code systems, which is still an international challenge due to lack of a unique international identifier for each active substance, dosage form and strength. In the system used by the hospitals in the Capital Region of Denmark the system on one hand cannot warn a nurse who dispenses the wrong form of a medicine – on the other hand if she dispenses another generic name than prescribed – she has to click away two warnings

7. Conclusion

Making good clinical decision support tools is a major challenge taken very seriously by all Danish stakeholders (public and private). The compulsory and anonymous reporting system driven by The Danish National Board of Health was a useful tool to identify potential high risk drugs and through a follow up process with clinicians it was possible to select relevant drugs. There is however no perfect coding system to import warnings into CPOE and decision support systems. Creating a unique international identifier for all active substances in a certain dosage form and strength would be an obvious improvement.

References

[1] Sundhedsstyrelsen. Temarapport om medicineringsfejl. 2005.
[2] Sundhedsstyrelsen. Temarapport om risikolægemidler. 2007.
[3] Medication Erros. APhA., 2007
[4] Rabøl, L., Hellebek, A., Pedersen A, Bredesen, J., and Lilja Beth. Elektronisk Beslutningsstøtte - en rapport. 2005. DLI og Dansk Selskab for Patientsikkerhed.
[5] Rabøl L, Hellebek A, Pedersen A, Bredesen J, Pedersen BL: Elektronisk beslutningsstøtte. Ugeskr Laeger 2006
[6] Lehmann M, Petersen ASJ, Hallas J, Hellebek A: Ordinationsfejl i Danmark. Ugeskr Laeger 2009
[7] Hellebek A: Medicineringsfejl. In www. medicin.dk. Infomatum, 2009

Detection and Prevention of Adverse Drug Events
R. Beuscart et al. (Eds.)
IOS Press, 2009

doi:10.3233/978-1-60750-043-8-32

ReMINE: An Ontology-based Risk Management Platform

Michele CARENINI [a, 1] and The ReMINE Consortium [2]
[a] *NoemaLife GmbH*

Abstract. The ReMINE project aims at building a high performance prediction, detection and monitoring platform for managing Risks against Patient Safety (RAPS). The project will contribute to the optimization of RAPS management process in a healthcare system through the development of a platform allowing the (semantically based) fast and secure extraction of RAPS-related data and their correlation across several domains. In this respect the REMINE platform will promote early RAPS detection and mitigation by supporting the process of RAPS management both when a RAPS is foreseen, and the objective is the determination of the best set of preventive actions; and when a RAPS is detected, and the objective is the determination of the best possible reaction, the reliable distribution of the related action list to all involved parties, and the monitoring of the reaction effectiveness. These capabilities will be achieved by means of the establishment of an associated methodology and a framework/platform for integrated RAPS prediction/detection, analysis and mitigation. The overall platform structure assumes the presence of an "info-broker patient safety framework" connected with the Hospital Information System, which will support the process of collecting, aggregating, mining and assessing related data, distributing alerts, and suggesting actions to mitigate (or avoid) RAPS effects or occurrence. The underlying ontological system will support the semantic correlation of data with the hospital processes.

Keywords. Patient Safety, Risk Management, Biomedical Ontologies, Decision Support System.

Introduction

Risks Against Patient Safety (RAPS) represent one of the most important causes of death in hospitals. In the phase of therapy, more than 8% of patients in the hospital suffer an additional disease due to RAPS. Almost 50% of the cases result to either death or significant additional health problems. RAPS occur in any stage of the patient care process; even if 50% of them are predictable, they are caused by the lack of proper communication amongst different actors of the patient care chain [1].

[1] Corresponding Author: Michele Carenini, NoemaLife GmbH, Alt-Moabit 96, 10559 Berlin, Germany; E-mail: mcarenini@noemalife.com.

[2] The ReMINE consortium is constituted by: Regione Lombardia, Direzione Generale Sanità (IT); Federation of Municipalities for Economic Development in Suupohja (FI); The Rotherham NHS Foundation Trust (UK); Hewlett-Packard Italiana Srl (IT); INDRA Slovakia, a.s. (CZ); Technische Universitaet Wien (AT); Research in Advanced Medical Informatics and Telematics (vzw) (BE); Quality & Reliability Sa – High Tech Applications Industrial & Commercial Societé Anonyme (GR); Link Consulting, Tecnologias e Sistemas de Informação, S.A. (POR); Institute of Communication and Computer Systems - National Technical University of Athens (GR); MIP Consorzio per l'innovazione e la Gestione delle Imprese e della Pubblica Amministrazione (IT); S.C. Info World S.R.L. (RO); AMINIO AB (SE).

Current approaches for RAPS early identification and effective prevention suffer from two major drawbacks: lack of RAPS information at the right time in the right place; and absence of standardized, easily accessible procedures. The ReMINE project[3] aims at the harmonization of RAPS detection and reaction methodologies through the identification of the main risk factors and the continuous revisions of the effectiveness and efficiency of the foreseen countermeasures. The ReMINE platform automated/semi-automated RAPS management and prevention relies on:

a) An effective RAPS identification and analysis through the acquisition and mining of relevant multimedia data from hospital care processes;
b) The use of results above for RAPS modelling, predicting and monitoring;
c) An efficient reaction procedure and the simultaneous involvement of different care professionals in a common risk management strategy.

The following paragraphs will focus on ReMINE architecture and how it integrates a number of AI techniques (decision support system, data mining, ontology); and on the system's taxonomy/ontology-based approach to Risk Management.

1. ReMINE Architecture

The data inserted into the system include hospital processes (mostly in paper format), electronic data from clinical devices, EHR data, RFID and Barcode data. All this information is transformed and filtered in a common format with the use of a structure modeling standard (XML, BPL and HL7) in order to obtain a semantic structure before entering the meta-database, where the domain classification (drug, lab, clinical pathways and patient management domain) is implemented.

After such semantic structuring, information is imported into the meta-database, containing the taxonomy and ontology sets and all the data in XML format, the existing processes, the new processes from the RAPS Process Model, knowledge from data mining and guidelines. The guidelines from the meta-database are transferred to the decision support system. These guidelines are formalized and, with the use of a guideline execution engine, eventually forwarded as output instructions to the RAPS Process Model. Data are inserted into the data mining module. This module performs knowledge extraction concerning possible risks in the hospital, and this knowledge is imported into the RAPS Process Model.

The RAPS Process Model platform is a graphical user interface which enables a business manager to work with business processes using Business Process Modeling methodologies and user-friendly notation (BPMN) [2,3]. More specifically, the user is able to design new processes, map, merge or update existing ones and execute business processes. The user can also evaluate "What-if" scenarios by modifying certain parameters, test a complete process or parts of it, and discover or define new risks through these trials. Moreover, a risk manager may design and configure risk alerts by creating and updating appropriate roles, actors and conditions. When a business process is executed, its activity is monitored and a Rule Engine evaluates risks according to

---

[3] ReMINE, "High Performance prediction, detection and monitoring platform for patient safety risk management" (Grant Agreement No. 216134), is an Integrated Project co-funded by the European Commission under the 7th Framework Programme (FP7/2007-2013).

rules created by the experts. This Rule engine cooperates with the taxonomy/ontology engine of the ReMINE system in order to correctly classify alerts and notifications and forward them, using Business Process Execution Language (BPEL) [4], to the respective Semantic Web Service wrapper engine. According to which domain the alert belongs to (drugs, lab, etc.), the corresponding wrapper is activated and sends an alert to the appropriate users. An alert output may also be produced and directed to the risk manager for evaluation purposes. The core of the RAPS Process Model relies on a Semantic Business Process Composer (SBPC), which administers all actions performed by the manager concerning the design, monitoring, evaluation and execution of business processes. Most parts of this mechanism are implemented through a modern business process management platform [5], which employs a performance reporting dashboard and can provide rule-based alerts and notifications. However, the RAPS Process Model is not only a business process management tool: it also admits information from the data mining and decision-support modules, therefore allowing the manager to monitor the corresponding guidelines concerning the current process and the results of the data mining component, since both aim at providing support to the manager to take proper decisions to reduce risk and improve patient safety.

1.1. The ReMINE Ontology as a System Component

Since the next paragraphs of this paper will deal mainly with the taxonomy/ontology component of the overall system, it may be worth summarizing how the such a component fits into the global ReMINE architecture.

The ReMINE ontology is primarily intended to represent a detailed domain description specifying relations between data events, identifying patient risks, and considering adverse events previously documented in the system. There is no “interface” with other components – the ontology needs to be “functionally integrated” into a number of components of the ReMINE application, namely:

- the *Process Mapper* component, to provide tags in the semantic structuring of the patient risk and safety management related processes;
- the *Data Event Management System*, in order to enrich/normalise the data passed-on from the *Data Acquisition Layer* and to improve the tagging of “data events”, allowing finally for the data to become searchable/retrievable by the *Data Mining* and/or *Knowledge Extraction* facilities;
- the *MetaDatabase Reasoner* in order to analyse “data events” to tag or semantically annotate data from the patient record and other sources as “adverse events”or “risks for adverse events”, and to check the semantic integrity of the incoming data before they are stored in the REMINE Database;
- the *Risk Manager Interface* component to represent patient safety adverse events and patient safety risks.

2. ReMINE Taxonomy/Ontology Approach to RAPS Management

Guidelines for care process aiming at the standardization of patient safety would greatly improve incident reporting, tracking, and analysis [6,7] and prevention. The ReMINE taxonomy can be considered as a building block for a multidimensional ontology, which in turn represents the knowledge base for the ReMINE decision support system.

2.1. ReMINE RAPS Taxonomy

First, a review of available taxonomies and standardized terminologies for risk management in healthcare has been carried out. One of the most relevant initiatives was the consultation document on the proposed establishment of core and developmental standards covering NHS healthcare provided for NHS patients published in February 2004 by the UK Dept. of Health [8]. This "Standard for a Risk Management System" has been recently updated to provide assistance in managing risks, hazards, incidents, complaints and claims, aiming at ensuring that all NHS organizations have the basic building blocks in place for managing risk. The ReMINE taxonomy takes profit from the definition of high-level general entities related to risk included in this standard. Besides NHS, two main reference taxonomies taken from most relevant initiatives carried out in the United States were selected: the JCAHO patient safety event taxonomy, a standardized terminology and classification schema for adverse events [9], and ICPS, the International Classification for Patient Safety, proposed by the World Health Organization [10], an attempt to identify a comprehensive classification of concepts with agreed definition. They both represented a useful resource for ReMINE taxonomy population. Web Ontology Language (OWL), the *de facto* standard for ontology engineering, was a natural choice.

2.2. ReMINE Dynamic Model

The distinction between "past events" and "events happening in a given setting", necessary to give account of the dynamic nature of risk prevention, has been made possible by introducing the concept of *Situation* in the *Adverse Event* taxonomy. The basic structure of the ReMINE taxonomy relies then on two concepts: *Situation*, composed by events occurring and being monitored (and feeding the ReMINE decision support system) during the patient staying in a hospital; and *Adverse_Event*, i.e. an incident occurred in the past and documented in a database.

The *Situation* refers to a particular healthcare process for a patient. It might present some *Risk Parameters* (e.g., staff over-commitment, negligent patient's behaviour) that can be similar to the *Contributing Factor* of past *Adverse_Events*. The Reasoning Module examines the current *Situation* interpreting risk factors and possibly recognizing *Risk Patterns*. If this is the case, the prevention system may decide to issue a warning and react to prevent risks against the patient. In addition, if *Risk Parameters* contributes to an adverse event, they are categorized as *Contributing Factors*, and the *Adverse_Event* database is consequently updated with the new incident. This allows to dynamically manage the risk situation and to enrich the knowledge about the incident type. In the ReMINE taxonomy the high level perspective of the JCHAO taxonomy was integrated with the main classes produced by ICPC standardization; concepts were contextualized in the SHEL model[4]:

---

[4] The SHEL model is composed by four components: Software (the non-physical aspects of the system such as procedures, protocols and guidelines), Hardware (all the physical aspects of the system such as medical devices, equipment and instruments), Environment (the specific settings, context within which an incident can occurs), and Liveware (all the aspects involving people and human factors and relationship) [11].

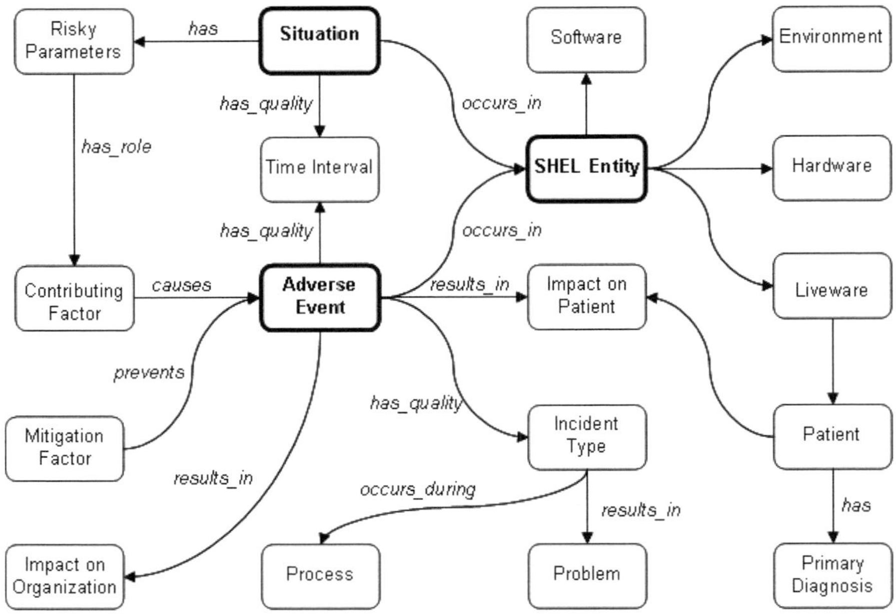

Figure 1. ReMINE Taxonomy Conceptual Scheme.

The central concept *Adverse_Event* has an impact both on the patient and on the organization (*Impact_on_Patient*, *Impact_on_Organization*). It occurs within a particular *Time_Interval* and in a given *SHEL* entity (e.g., a given medical unit, a surgeon, a given medical device and an operating theatre). A relevant concept for describing the incident is the *Incident_Type*, decomposed along two dimensions: the *Process* during which the incident occurs (e.g., patient identification, test, dispensing nutrition); and the *Problem* that occurred (e.g., wrong patient identification, test not performed when due, wrong nutrition quantity dispensed). The *Adverse_Event* may have *Contributing Factors* that cause the incident and *Mitigation Factors* that can prevent the incident. It may be worth stressing the fact that the main approach within ReMINE has been that of developing a general framework in order to represent the main aspects of the RAPS domain, preserving the possibility to extend it in order to capture peculiar aspects of specific healthcare domains. For instance, the general *Impact_on_Patient* class has been specialized to the *Specific_Gynaecological_Impact* [12]. Such an approach proved to be particularly suitable for updating, enlarging and expanding iteratively the proposed taxonomy.

3. Basic Assumptions in Taxonomies and Ontologies Design

One basic choice to be taken when designing taxonomies and ontologies deals with the notion of *change*, i.e. answering the question “What does it mean for an entity to change?”. Such a question raises the problem of variation in time and the related issue of identity of objects.

In general a 3D option claims that objects are:

a) Extended in a three dimensional space;

b) Wholly present at each instant of their existence;
c) Changing entities, in the sense that at different times they can instantiate different properties.

A four dimensional perspective, instead, states that objects are:

a) Space-time worms;
b) Only partially present at each instant;
c) Changing entities, in the sense that at different phases they can have different properties.

The DOLCE ("Descriptive Ontology for Linguistic and Cognitive Engineering", [13]) foundational ontology contains a description of the basic kinds of entities and relationships that are assumed to exist in some domain, such as *process*, *object*, *time*, *part*, *location*, *representation*, etc. DOLCE is a 3D cognitively-oriented ontology, based on primitive space and time, distinguishing between objects and processes as well as between physical and intentional objects. DOLCE is defined as a descriptive ontology since it is used to categorize an already existing conceptualization: DOLCE does not state *how* things are, but how they can be represented according to some existing knowledge.

Basic elements of DOLCE are:

- *Endurants* (aka *Continuants*), classically characterized as entities "wholly present" (i.e. all their proper parts are present) at any time of their existence;
- *Perdurants* (aka *Occurrents*), entities that "happen in time", extending in time by accumulating different "temporal parts" – at any time *t* where they exist, only their temporal parts at *t* are present;
- *Qualities*, the basic entities that can be perceived or measured – shapes, colors, sizes, sounds, smells, weights, lengths, etc.

Endurants and perdurants can be characterized in a different way: something is an endurant if (i) it exists at more than one moment, and (ii) its parts can be determined only in relation with something else (e.g., time). In other words, the distinction is based on the fact that endurants need a time-indexed parthood, while perdurants do not.[5]

In the context of the ReMINE basic taxonomy, endurants like *Problem*, *SHEL entity*, *Contributing factor*, *Mitigation factor* were identified; dynamic concepts as *Process* and *Adverse event* represent perdurants; *Time interval* and *Incident type* are examples of qualities.

4. Operational Strategy for ReMINE Taxonomy Development

The ReMINE taxonomy development has been conceived to provide continuous support to the lifecycle management of the developed ontology. For this reason a continuous process has been followed, through which the taxonomy can be validated, updated, modified and evaluated by experts. Figure 2 shows the development lifecycle for ReMINE taxonomy.

---

[5] Compare a statement like "This keyboard is part of my computer" (which is incomplete unless a particular time is specified) to "My youth is part of my life" (which does not require a time specification).

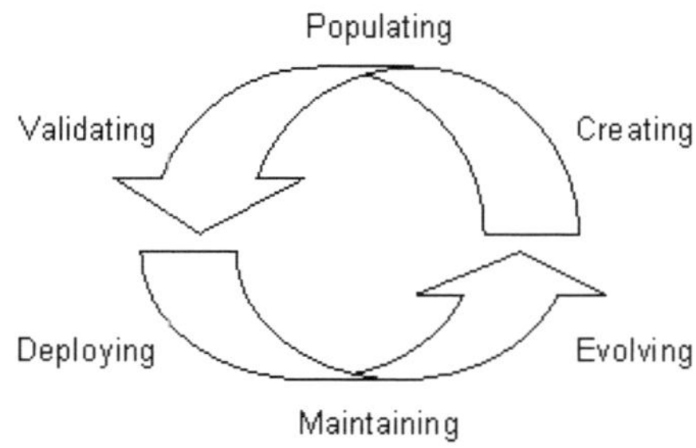

Figure 2. ReMINE Development Lifecycle.

“Creating” is the initial phase where the backbone taxonomy has been developed and the general approach has been decided. The collaborative work with domain experts and the feedback from ontology engineers allowed to validate the taxonomy and approve the general approach. The process, then, continues iteratively through a deeper involvement of domain experts and feedback collection from pilots, thus allowing “Maintaining”, and allowing for the initial ReMINE framework evolution in order to make it more suitable for specific real applications needs. Such an iterative process will guarantee a continuous support to the lifecycle of the ReMINE ontology.

In order to adopt one most effective and sharable development process, a strategy based on Method, Model and Standard (MMS) has been chosen.

4.1. Method

In order to capture the main relevant aspects of the RAPS domain, the approach adopted to design the ReMINE taxonomy produced a general backbone of the whole representation allowing for the addition of extensions driven by pilot sites – case studies related to different medical units. Within ReMINE, the focus was put onto areas that are particularly sensitive to the risk of serious accidents.

In fact a key point in ReMINE is to focus on a selection of pilots in areas which are particularly relevant with respect to the risk of serious incidents. Hence the development of the specific taxonomy and related ontology domain for risk factors and related RAPS classification and correlation is made through the interactive involvement of ontology engineers and the pilot domain experts in a continuous refinement process. As an example specific terms related to the *Gynaecological domain*, the Str*oke unit* and the *Geriatrics domain* have been added to highlight how the general structure can be extended and modified according to the needs of the chosen pilots. In order to develop both the general taxonomy and specific terms of the pilots, state-of-the-art taxonomies were merged with input coming from particular clinical domain experts. The taxonomy can be continuously refined and updated when new input from domain experts is received.

4.2. Model

The first phase of the project included the analysis of the state of the art in terms of risk management and the exploitation of ontology engineering. Some existing relevant projects have been identified, and possibilities to take them into account within ReMINE have been evaluated.

4.3. Standard

The next decision concerned the way to represent the taxonomy, as well as the kind of tool to be used for supporting its development. Since one main aspect of ReMINE is its re-usability in different domains and though different platforms, standard technology for the development of the taxonomy content has been chosen – Web Ontology Language (OWL).[6]

5. The ReMINE Development Method

As previously described, the development of the specific RAPS taxonomy was based on the interactive involvement of ontology engineers and domain experts, who contributed to the realization of a general framework capturing the main relevant aspects of the RAPS domain.

5.1. Main Entities of the ReMINE Taxonomy

In accordance with the DOLCE foundational ontology, the backbone of the ReMINE taxonomy has been designed according to the Endurant, Perdurant, and Quality classification.

Endurants include:

- *Primary_Diagnosis*, a primary diagnosis of a patient;
- *Impact_on_Organization*, the possible impact that an Adverse Event can have on the organization;
- *Mitigation_Factor*, an action or circumstance which prevents or moderates the progression of an *Adverse_Event* and the relative impact on the patient or on the organization;
- *Contributing Factor*, an action or circumstance which can play a part in the origin or development of an Adverse_Event, or increase the risk of an incident[7];
- *Problem*, representing what actually occurred to the patient;
- *SHEL Entity*, representing the combination of *Software*, *Hardware*, *Environmental* and *Liveware aspects*, settings or problems that are used to describe an *Adverse_Event*;
- *Impact_on_Patient*, indicating the impact that an *Adverse_Event* has on the patient;
- *Risky_Parameters*, indicating dangerous patterns that are recognized as possible responsible for an *Adverse_Event*.

The Perdurant elements consists of the following terms:

---

[6] OWL is a W3C endorsed format that can be used to define relatively rich semantics and system of hierarchical types, which can be used to describe entities.

[7] The *Contributing Factor* is subdivided according to the SHEL Model into: *Software_Contributing_Factor*, *Hardware_Contributing_Factor*, *Environment_Contributing_Factor* and *Liveware_Contributing_Factor*.

- *Process*, during which the incident occurs (e.g., Patient identification, test, dispensing nutrition, etc.);
- *Adverse_Event*, the incident that occurred to a patient;
- *Situation*, the current situation that is to be monitored in order to prevent adverse events.

The Quality elements are constituted by:

- *Time_Interval* during which an adverse event can occur;
- *Patient_Quality*, as, e.g., age, gender;
- *Degree_of_Harm* with five possible values: *Death*, *Severe*, *Moderate*, *Mild*, *None*;
- *Incident_Type*, which can be extended and expanded so as to capture different domains.

5.2. Extending the ReMINE Taxonomy

As already mentioned, one main priority in the development of ReMINE was to preserve the possibility to extend the general framework in order to capture the peculiar aspects of specific healthcare domains. All classes of the taxonomy can be iteratively expanded. Figure 3 represents the insertion of *Specific_Gynaecological_Impact* into the *Impact_on_Patient* class:

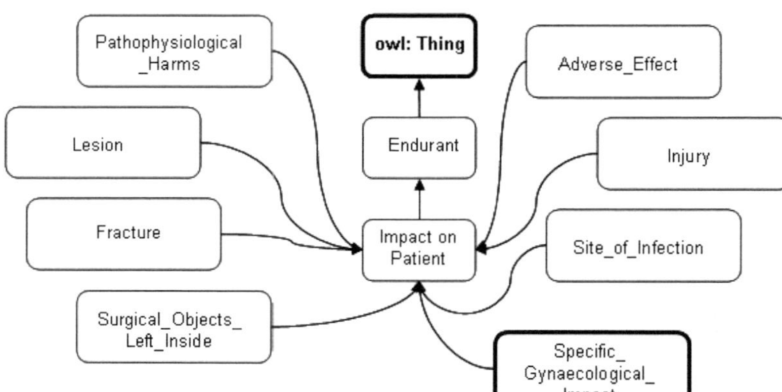

Figure 3. Extension to capture one pilot domain specificity.

While figure 4 shows the specialization of the *Impact_on_Patient* class through the full instantiation of *Specific_Gynaecological_Impact*:

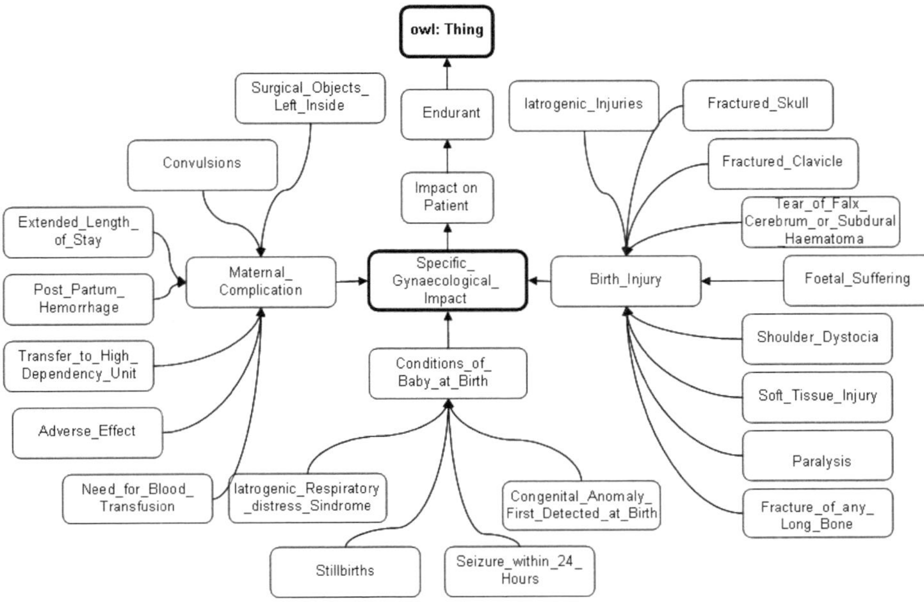

Figure 4. Specific Gynaecological Impact Main Classes.

6. Conclusions

After one year ReMINE achieved a number of goals, including the design and development of the taxonomy backbone for RAPS and the specialization of specific domains ontologies. Being an ongoing project, many tasks need to be performed and completed. One of the most important ones is the further development of the application ontology underlying the RAPS taxonomy. Focus on pilot applications will take to possible application ontologies to be implemented throughout the lifecycle of the project. The choice of the representation language to be used represent another main challenge for the continuation of the project. The one that is selected will have both to comply to *de facto* standards and provide mechanisms to manage temporal aspects of instantiation.

Acknowledgments

This paper is significantly based on a number of ReMINE deliverables, in particular: D4.1, "RAPS Taxonomy: approach and definition" (main contributing partner: MIP Consorzio per l'innovazione e la Gestione delle Imprese e della Pubblica Amministrazione – IT), D4.2, "RAPS Domain Ontology" (main contributing partner: Research in Advanced Medical Informatics and Telematics vzw – BE), and D6.1, "ReMINE Architecture Specifications" (main contributing partner: Quality & Reliability Sa – GR). Preliminary versions of this paper have been read and commented by Gianpiero Camilli, Sebastiano Amoddio, Cristiano Querzè, Massimo Vanocchi at

NoemaLife. ReMINE is a project co-funded by the European Commission (Project No. 216134) under the 7th Framework Programme (FP7/2007-2013).

References

[1] M. Woloshynowych, C. Vincent, Exploring the causes of adverse events in NHS hospital practice, J. Soc. Med. 94 (2001), 322–330.

[2] M. Owen, J. Raj, BPMN and Business Process Management: Introduction to the New Business Process Modeling Standard, Popkin Software White Paper, 2003.

[3] Object Management Group, Business Process Modeling Notation (BPMN) Specification, Final Adopted Specification, 2006.

[4] B. Margolis, J. Sharp, SOA for the Business Developer: Concepts, BPEL, and SCA (Business Developers series), MC Press, Double Oak, 2007.

[5] IDS Scheer, ARIS Process Performance Manager (ARIS PPM), http://www.idsscheer.com.

[6] Quality Interagency Coordination Task Force (QuIC): Doing What Counts for Patient Safety: Federal Actions to Reduce Medical Errors and Their Impact. Report to the President. http://www.quic.gov/report/toc.htm (2000).

[7] H. Kaplan, J.B. Battles, T.W. Van der Schaaf, C.E. Shea, S.Q. Mercer, Identification and classification of the causes of events in transfusion medicine. Transfusion 38 (1998), 1071–1081.

[8] University of Westminster, School of Integrated Health, Risk Management in Health Care, http://www.wmin.ac.uk/sih/page-568.

[9] A. Chang, P.M. Schyve, R.J. Croteau, D.S. O'Leary, J.M. Loeb, The JCAHO patient safety event taxonomy: a standardized terminology and classification schema for near misses and adverse events, Int. J. Qual. Health Care 17(2) (2005), 92–105.

[10] World Health Organization, International Classification for Patient Safety (ICPS). http://www.who.int/patientsafety/taxonomy/en/.

[11] G.J. Molloy, C.A. O'Boyle, The SHEL model: a useful tool for analyzing and teaching the contribution of Human Factors to medical error. Acad. Med. 80(2), (2005) 152–155.

[12] S. Arici, P. Bertelè, RAPS Taxonomy: approach and definition, ReMINE Project 216134, Deliverable 4.1 (2008).

[13] A. Gangemi, N. Guarino, C. Masolo, A. Oltramari, L. Schneider, Sweetening Ontologies with DOLCE, Proceedings of the 13th European Conference on Knowledge Engineering and Knowledge Management (EKAW2002), Siguenza, Spain, 2002.

Detection and Prevention of Adverse Drug Events
R. Beuscart et al. (Eds.)
IOS Press, 2009

doi:10.3233/978-1-60750-043-8-43

The EU-ADR Project: Preliminary Results and Perspective

Gianluca TRIFIRO [a, b, 1], Annie FOURRIER-REGLAT [c], Miriam C.J.M. STURKENBOOM [a], Carlos DÍAZ ACEDO [d] and Johan VAN DER LEI [a], on behalf of the EU-ADR Group

[a] *Department of Medical Informatics, Erasmus University Medical Center, Rotterdam, The Netherlands*
[b] *IRCCS Centro Neurolesi ''Bonino-Pulejo'', Messina, Italy*
[c] *Inserm U 657, Pharmacology Department, Bordeaux, France*
[d] *Fundació IMIM - European Projects Management Office, Barcelona, Spain.*

Abstract. The EU-ADR project aims to exploit different European electronic healthcare records (EHR) databases for drug safety signal detection. In this paper we describe the project framework and the preliminary results. Methods: As first step we created a ranked list of the events that are deemed to be important in pharmacovigilance as mining on all possible events was considered to unduly increase the number of spurious signals. All the drugs that are potentially associated to these events will be detected via data mining techniques. Data sources are eight 8 databases in four countries (Denmark, Italy, the Netherlands, and the United Kingdom) that are virtually linked through harmonisation of input data followed by local elaboration of input data through custom-built software (Jerboa©). All the identified drug-event associations (signals) will be thereafter biologically substantiated and epidemiologically validated. To date, only Upper gastrointestinal bleeding (UGIB) event has been used to test the ability of the system in signal detection. Results: An initial ranked list comprising 23 adverse events was identified. The top-ranking events were: cutaneous bullous eruptions, acute renal failure, acute myocardial infarction, anaphylactic shock, and rhabdomyolysis. Regarding the UGIB test, a total of 48,016 first-ever episodes were identified. The age-standardized incidence rates of UGIB varied between 40-100/100,000 person-years depending on country and type of healthcare database. A statistically significant association between use of NSAIDs and UGIB was detected in all of the databases. Conclusion: a dynamic ranked list of 23 adverse drug events judged as important in pharmacovigilance was created to permit focused data mining. Preliminary results on the UGIB event detection demonstrate the feasibility of harmonizing various health care databases in different European countries through a distributed network approach.

Keywords: Pharmacovigilance, electronic health records, biomedical knowledge, signal generation, signal substantiation

Introduction

In pharmacovigilance, a signal is defined by the World Health Organization as information on a possible causal relationship between an adverse event and a drug,

1 Corresponding Author: trifirog@unime.it

which is unknown or incompletely documented. [1,2] Spontaneous reporting systems for adverse drug reactions (ADRs) have been the cornerstone of signal detection in pharmacovigilance for the last four decades.[3,4] However, it has become evident that some adverse effects of drugs may be detected too late, when millions of persons have already been exposed. The increasing availability of electronic healthcare records (EHRs) presents opportunities to investigate a wide spectrum of adverse drug effects and to detect signals closer to real time. [5,6] Compared to data from clinical trials, data from EHR databases reflect better situations in actual clinical practice where drugs are used by a more diverse patient population. [7] In addition EHR databases offer the additional advantage of large populations and long follow-up periods. A number of data mining techniques have been specifically developed for automatic detection of drug safety signals [3].

It is within this context of exploring the use of EHRs as an adjunct to drug safety monitoring that the EU-ADR project was conceived. EU-ADR, "Exploring and Understanding Adverse Drug Reactions by integrative mining of clinical records and biomedical knowledge (EU-ADR)" (http://www.euadr-project.org), is a project funded by the European Commission, which began in February 2008. The overall objective of the project is to design, develop, and validate a computerized integrative system that exploits data from EHRs and biomedical databases for the early detection of ADRs. Beyond the current state-of-the-art, EU-ADR led to the federation of different databases of EHRs, creating a resource of unprecedented size for drug safety monitoring in Europe (over 30 million patients from eight different databases). The initial stage of signal generation will be followed by signal substantiation through causal reasoning, semantic mining of literature, and computational analysis of pharmacological and biological information, all with the aim of finding possible pathways that explain the drug-event associations (Figure 1).

As regard signal generation, in the EU-ADR project we used an event-based approach where a set of specific events are inspected for their association with all possible drugs. One of the challenges in the event-based approach to signal detection through mining on EHR databases is the identification of events that are most important in pharmacovigilance and thus warrant priority for monitoring. Indeed, unconstrained data mining is likely to raise excessive numbers of spurious signals. For this reason, the first task of this project was to create a ranked list of high-priority events from a pharmacovigilance perspective. This list of events shall be the starting point for signal detection in the EU-ADR project.

The aim of the current paper is to describe the main project framework and to present the preliminary results of the EU-ADR project. In particular, the ranked list of events and the first results on the query harmonization across eight different electronic health record databases, using the event Upper Gastrointestinal Bleeding (UGIB), will be briefly reported.

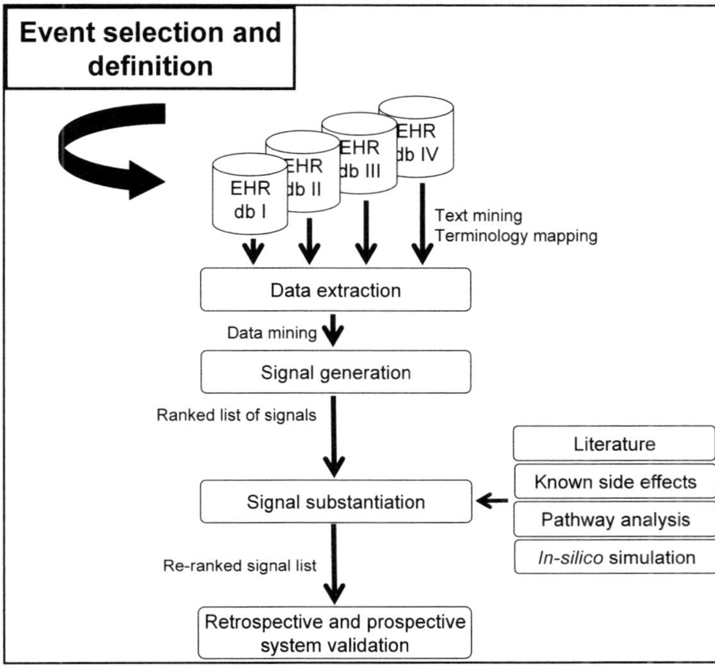

Figure 1. Overview of the EU-ADR data management and processing. Data are extracted and aggregated from the participating EHR databases. Data mining tools are used for signal generation. These signals are substantiated using causal reasoning and biomedical knowledge, and thereafter assessed to evaluate the system's capabilities.

1. Methods

The EU-ADR project platform consist of a network of electronic medical record databases from different European countries: IPCI and PHARMO (Netherlands), QRESEARCH (UK), the AUHD database (Denmark), the Regional health databases of Lombardy and Tuscany, Health Search/Thales and PEDIANET (Italy). After the identification of a ranked list of events, automated signal generation will be conducted by applying data mining techniques on data from the eight databases. All the identified pairs of drug-event that represent possible signals will be thereafter substantiated by computer-assisted exploration of their biological plausibility in the context of current biomedical knowledge with the final aim to reduce the false positive signals. Finally, all the potential signals that are refined and substantiated will be validated by undertaking traditional epidemiologic investigations.

To date, the main activities of the project focused on the creation of prioritized list of events and on the query harmonization for the detection of UGIB event and possible association with non steroidal anti-inflammatory drug exposure. This combination of class drug-event was primarily considered to test the sensitivity of the EU-ADR system in detecting well-known associations.

Both in the methods and the results section we only described the two above-mentioned tasks.

1.1. Creation of a ranked list of events

For the priority event selection and ranking, a four-step procedure was outlined by two teams of 4 pharmacovigilance experts each, from two institutions (Department of Pharmacology and Regional Pharmacovigilance Centre at the Université Victor-Segalen in Bordeaux, France, and the IRCCS Centro Neurolesi "Bonino Pulejo", Messina, Italy).

Step 1: Identification of important events

A list of important adverse drug events was compiled, considering different system/organ classes. These events were identified from pharmacovigilance reference books and publications reviewing reasons for drug withdrawal and from information on websites of drug regulatory agencies.

Step 2: Creation of a criteria set for event rating

To rank the events according to public health importance, five criteria were considered: 1) Frequency of the event as trigger for drug withdrawal; 2) Frequency of the event as trigger for black box warning; 3) Leading to emergency department visit or hospital admission; 4) Probability of event to be drug-related; and 5) Likelihood of death. For each criterion, ordinal scales were defined ranging from 0 (irrelevant) to 3 (highly relevant).

Step 3: Score assignment

The two pharmacovigilance teams independently assigned scores for each of the events. Scores were based on a comprehensive review of the scientific literature over the past 10 years and the evaluation of other sources of information. In case of disagreement about a score, consensus was obtained after discussion among all members of the two teams.

Step 4: Ranking of events

For each event, an overall score was computed by summing up the five criteria scores. Based on the overall scores, a ranked event list was made. The top-ranked events were considered as having the highest priority for drug safety monitoring.

1.2. UGIB event query harmonization

The EU-ADR project has chosen a common data model to create harmonized input files from the databases. These input files are created locally and are subsequently queried by a purpose-built software called Jerboa© to aggregate the data across the different databases. Database owners run the software locally and maintain complete control of the security of their respective data. The resulting summarized and encrypted data is then sent to a central repository for evaluation and analysis.

Jerboa© requires three Input files containing information on patient (patient identifier, gender, age, start and end of eligibility), drugs (patient identifier, date of dispensing/prescription, ATC code, and duration) and events (patient identifier, type of event and date of event). Common definitions have been provided to harmonize the information that is provided by each database. The first event that has been tested was Upper Gastrointestinal Bleeding (UGIB). Differences exists in coding schemes and terminologies («international statistical classification of diseases and related health problems» (ICD9-CM and ICD10), the «international classification of primary care» (ICPC) and the READ CODE (RCD) classification) that are used to register the diagnosis of UGIB among medical record databases. The different terminologies have been mapped using the The Unified Medical Language System® (UMLS®).

After generating the three input files (patient, drug and UGIB event), Jerboa© queried and aggregated the data over all patients locally, outputting person-time, and events per age group and gender. In such a way, we first calculated the crude incidence rates of UGIB, stratified by age and gender, per database and in aggregated way.

As second step, we used Jerboa© for the estimation of risk of the event associated with NSAID exposure. Analyses have been done at three ATC levels: pharmacological subgroup (e.g., M01A); chemical subgroup (e.g., M01AB, M01AC, etc); and chemical substance (e.g., M01AC01). Relative risks are calculated using the Mantel-Haenszel method.

2. Results

2.1. Ranked list of events

Twenty-three events were identified in the first step of the event selection process. These were classified by organ/body system into: hematologic; cutaneous; liver and gastrointestinal; cardiac and vascular; neurologic; psychiatric; renal; and multi-systemic. On the basis of the overall scores, the top-ranked events were: cutaneous bullous eruptions, acute renal failure, acute myocardial infarction, anaphylactic shock, and rhabdomyolysis.

As an example, cutaneous bullous eruption (Stevens-Johnson syndrome or Lyell's syndrome) emerged as one of the most important events, garnering a score of 15 points: at least 5 drugs have been withdrawn from the market due to this adverse reaction, viz., valdecoxib, chlormezanone, sulfamethoxypyridazine, sulfadimethoxine, and isoxicam, and multiingredients preparations containing phenobarbital (criterion "trigger for drug withdrawal", 3 points); a black box warning for risk of cutaneous bullous reactions has been imposed on more than 10 drugs ("trigger for black box warning", 3 points); more than 5 papers have reported this adverse event as being responsible for emergency department visit or hospitalization ("leading to emergency department visit or hospital admission", 3 points); at least 70% of cutaneous bullous reactions have been attributed to drug exposure ("probability of event to be drug-related", 3 points); more than 30% of Stevens-Johnson/Lyell's syndrome cases are fatal, mainly because of progression to sepsis or pulmonary involvement ("likelihood of death", 3 points).

2.2. Upper Gastrointestinal Bleeding event detection

Almost 30 millions of individuals from all eight databases comprised the total study population, corresponding to about 60 million person-years of follow-up. Comparison of demographic profiles across databases reveal similar age and gender distributions (except for Pedianet which only includes patients aged less than 14 years and Health Search which covers patients older than 14 years old).

A total of 48,016 first-time episodes of UGIB, regardless of etiology, were identified using the queries defined by each database. Analysis of crude incidence rates demonstrate heterogeneity across the different databases, with rates of UGIB ranging from 39.1 (PHARMO) to 57.4 (IPCI) in the Netherlands to 108.6 (Aarhus) and 110.5

(Health Search) in Denmark and Italy, respectively. Incidence rates for the UK database (QRESEARCH) and the regional Italian databases (Tuscany and Lombardy) are somewhere in between. Comparison of age-standardized incidence rates shows an attenuation of this variation, although the rates for Aarhus remain high.

A bimodal pattern of UGIB is shown in all databases with respect to increasing age. An initial, but much smaller, peak occurs in the very young (0-4 years) with incidence rates of up to 30 per 100,000 person-years. Rates remain relatively stable in adolescence until late adulthood, but begin to rise again gradually in the fifth decade of life. The relative risk for UGIB in individuals 80 years and older is 14 times greater compared to those aged 40-49 years old (13.6, 14.7). Males appear to have a slightly increased risk for UGIB compared to females (RR 1.25 [1.23, 1.27]), with this difference becoming more pronounced from the sixth decade of life onwards.

A statistically significant ($p <<< 0.01$) risk for UGIB with the use of NSAIDs was found in all the 8 databases, despite a wide variation in the use of individual classes of NSAIDs among the databases, especially with respect to the COX-2 specific inhibitors and other NSAIDs like nimesulide, which is only available in some countries in Europe. Use of any NSAID conferred a crude relative risk (age- and gender-adjusted) for UGIB at least double that of non-NSAID use. Analysis of specific NSAID classes likewise show, more or less, consistent relative risk estimates across databases with COX-2 inhibitors exhibiting the lowest risk.

3. Conclusion

EU-ADR develops new integrative methods for exploiting electronic health care databases of more than 30 million Europeans plus existing biomedical knowledge, for faster detection and substantiation of drug safety signals. Data mining and computational tools have been used and will be further developed to discover and understand important drug safety signals.

To date, prioritization of adverse events judged as important in pharmacovigilance was undertaken to optimize data mining and to contain the number of spurious signals that data mining on EHR databases may generate. The focus of signal detection in the EU-ADR project will be a list of 23 ranked events, in which the top-ranking events were cutaneous bullous eruptions, acute renal failure, acute myocardial infarction, anaphylactic shock, and rhabdomyolysis.

Additionally, using the Upper Gastrointestinal bleeding event as test, our preliminary results demonstrated the feasibility of harmonizing various health care databases in different European countries through a distributed network approach. This approach allows for pooling of aggregated data and is expandable to accommodate other data sources in Europe, and eventually other parts of the world, to enlarge the scale for drug safety monitoring.

Acknowledgment

This research has been funded by the European Commission Seventh Framework Programme (FP7/2007-2013) under grant no. 215847 – The EU-ADR Project.

References

[1] M. Stahl, I.R. Edwards, G. Bowring, et al. Assessing the impact of drug safety signals from the WHO database presented in "SIGNAL'': results from a questionnaire of National Pharmacovigilance Centres. Drug Saf 26 (2003), 721-7.

[2] The Uppsala Monitoring Centre. Practical Pharmacovigilance. Signal Definition. http://www.who-umc.org/DynPage.aspx?id=22676#signaldef (accessed 5 February, 2009).

[3] E.M. Rodriguez, J.A. Staffa, D.J. Graham. The role of databases in drug postmarketing surveillance. Pharmacoepidemiol Drug Saf 10 (2001), 407-10.

[4] R.H.B. Meyboom, M. Lindquist, A.C.G. Egberts, et al. Signal detection and follow-up in pharmacovigilance. Drug Saf 25 (2002), 459–465.

[5] S. Schneeweiss and J. Avorn. A review of uses of health care utilization databases for epidemiologic research on therapeutics. J Clin Epidemiology 58 (2005), 323-37.

[6] J.S. Brown, M. Kulldorff, K.A. Chan, et al. Early detection of adverse drug events within population-based health networks: application of sequential testing methods. Pharmacoepidemiol Drug Saf 16 (2007), 1275-84.

[7] J.P. Vandenbroucke and B.M. Psaty. Benefits and risks of drug treatments: how to combine the best evidence on benefits with the best data about adverse effects. JAMA 300 (2008), 2417-9.

Detection and Prevention of Adverse Drug Events
R. Beuscart et al. (Eds.)
IOS Press, 2009

doi:10.3233/978-1-60750-043-8-50

DebugIT: Building a European Distributed Clinical Data Mining Network to Foster the Fight Against Microbial Diseases

Christian LOVIS [a, 1], Teodoro DOUGLAS [a], Emilie PASCHE [a], Patrick RUCH [a], Dirk COLAERT [b], and Karl STROETMANN [c]
[a] *University Hospitals of Geneva, Switzerland*
[b] *Agfa HealthCare, Belgium*
[c] *empirica GmbH, Germany*
for the DebugIT consortium

Abstract. The expansion of clinical information systems and the reduction in computing costs have led to an explosion of patient data available for reuse. However, this data is rarely combined and analyzed in an integrated manner. The DebugIT project is a large-scale integrating project funded within the 7th EU Framework Programme (FP7). The main objectives of the project are to build IT tools that should have significant impacts for the monitoring and the control of infectious diseases and antimicrobial resistances in Europe; this will be realized by building a technical and semantic infrastructure able to a) share heterogeneous clinical data sets from different hospitals in different countries, with different languages and legislations; b) analyze large amounts of this clinical data with advanced multi-modal data mining; c) apply the obtained knowledge for clinical decisions and outcome monitoring. The concepts and architecture underlying this project are discussed.

Keywords. Infectious disease, patient safety, semantic inter-operability, multi-modal data mining, decision support, clinical outcome monitoring

Introduction

Building a safer and more efficient care system has become the most shared goal of all actors involved in healthcare. From a historical perspective, there has been an impressive shift towards awareness of the impact of errors in medicine in the last 25 years. In the early nineties, research papers and reports about patient safety, incident reporting and initial order-entry systems were published, mostly originating from academic settings. At about the same time, the first reports of the US Institute of Medicine (IOM) on computerized patient record systems stressed the ability of ICT-based solutions to improve the quality of care [1]. Ten years later, by the end of the nineties, a famous report of the IOM called attention to the wide prevalence of errors in healthcare [2]. While medical errors are under the spotlight, (re-)emerging infectious diseases are becoming major challenges. Among them, the rapid development of anti-

[1] Corresponding Author: Service of Medical Informatics, University Hospitals of Geneva; E-mail: Christian.lovis@hcuge.ch

microbial resistances [3], the spread of nosocomial and other infections [4], the inadequate care and missing appropriate tools to lead the care system facing these new emergent problems [5] are major concerns. The issues around infectious diseases are strongly interrelated and have immediate and important effects on safety, quality of care and efficiency. In half a century of antibiotic use, new challenges have emerged: fast emergence of resistances among pathogens, misuse and overuse of antibiotics. Antimicrobial resistance results in escalating healthcare costs, increased morbidity and mortality and the (re-) emergence of potentially untreatable pathogens.

1. The Project

Dedicated to infectious diseases, the DebugIT (Detecting and Eliminating Bacteria UsinG Information Technology) project aims at (1) detecting patient safety related patterns and trends, (2) acquiring new knowledge and (3) using this for better quality healthcare. A consortium of eleven partners has been built in order to gather scientific competencies in all domains involved, as well as to assure access to specific information of more than 2 million clinical records.

Table 1. Consortium

Belgium	Agfa HealthCare
Bulgaria	GAMA/SOFIA Ltd.
Czech Republic	IZIP - Internetový Přistup Ke Zdravotním Informacím Pacienta
France	Institut National de la Santé et de la Recherche Médicale (with European Hospital George Pompidou) (INSERM)
Germany	empirica GmbH
Germany	University Medical Center Freiburg (UKLFR)
Greece	Technological Educational Institute of Lamia
Sweden	Linköping University (LIU)
Switzerland	University Hospital of Geneva (HUG)
Switzerland	University of Geneva, Computer Science Department
United Kingdom	University College London

The project has a strong clinical lead guaranteed by a Clinical Advisory Board and a Scientific Advisory Board with European and American experts of the infectiology field and the scientific domains involved.

Outcomes and benefits, in clinical and socio-economic terms, will be measured. Clinical results will be integrated into Clinical Information Systems (CIS) of participating European hospitals, industry and their clients, and become available globally through a European or global Disease Control Centre/Public Authority, also as Open Source solution. Advanced ICT applications and innovations concern the virtualization of the Clinical Data Repository through ontology and terminology binding and mediation, advanced data mining techniques, the use of machine reasoning related to real, point-of-care patient data, as well as consolidation of all these techniques in a comprehensive but open framework. Output will be applicable to other clinical fields.

The comprehensive concept, developed from such considerations as foundation for the DebugIT project, addresses all of these issues in an operational manner with the ultimate goal to develop a new, highly advanced and pre-eminent tool aiming at producing a new and efficient weapon for the war against infectious pathogens across all health system actors and levels.

The overall project outcome will not only be a theoretical work and proof of concept, but also a practical implementation of a highly improved and advanced computerised system in the field of infectious disease treatment and antibiotics usage. This application, which, due to its generic conceptual base, should be easily expandable and adaptable to other similar medical application fields, will initially be evaluated by participating project partners, but should be made publicly available to other healthcare organizations soon after.

2. The Conceptual Framework

The conceptual framework of this project is an ever continuing iterative cycle, implementing the principle of translational medicine and true Evidence Based Medicine (EBM). Translational medicine makes the connection between medical research and clinical care by providing to research clinical data and providing the results of the research – the medical knowledge – as input for clinical care. While medical research is often focusing on prospective and tightly controlled studies, retrospective studies with access to huge amounts of data, just waiting to be analyzed, are a welcome addition to clinical research.

The framework can be broken down into several distinct steps:

Collect Data. Clinical data will be collected and aggregated across different hospitals, countries, languages, information models and legislations, via advanced and commonly agreed data models (minimal data sets), standards and mapping algorithms.

Learn: Advanced data mining techniques on multimodal, multi-source, structured and unstructured data will detect patterns, relevant for patient safety and the treatment of infectious diseases such as: resistance of bacteria, adverse events and operational practices. This will result in new knowledge and new evidences for existing knowledge.

Store Knowledge: This knowledge will be stored, visualized, validated and aggregated together with pre-existing medical and biological knowledge (guidelines, regulations) to achieve a consolidated view on the needed knowledge, to be applied in the next step.

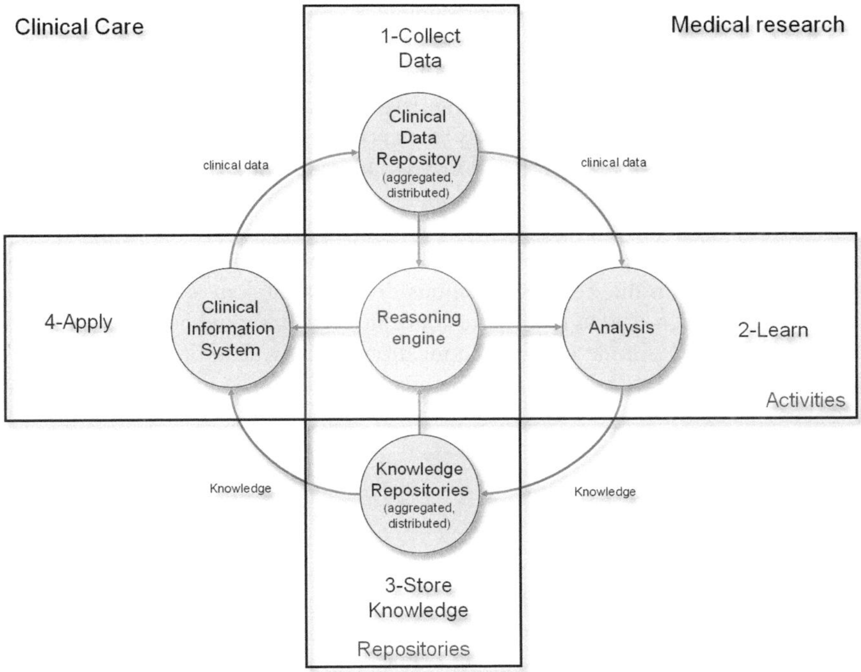

Figure 1. The Conceptual Framework

Apply: Software tools will be integrated into the available clinical and public health information systems. Decision support tools will apply the generated knowledge and help the clinician to provide clinical care (choice, dose and administration of antibiotics for example). The knowledge will also be used to monitor the ongoing care activities and even predict future outcome to give additional feedback, both on individual patient and cohort level. This will allow healthcare providers and decision makers to take appropriate actions at various levels of the healthcare system, including point-of-care, management or policy, and subsequently influence the future development of our health systems. Integration in existing CIS will enable to record activities and results and thus make sure the necessary data are generated for a next cycle.

3. Technology and Architecture

To achieve its goals, the DebugIT project will make extensive use of clinical and operational information originating from running Clinical Information Systems (CIS) across the EU, building a virtualized, fully integrated Clinical Data Repository (CDR).

The CDR will feature transparent access to the original CIS and provide data aggregations in local stores. The CDR is specifically tailored for knowledge discovery, featuring ethically sound, transparent access to data at or from the original CIS and/or collection and aggregation of data in a local data store.

Multimodal Data Mining (MDM) will have a strong focus on new fields of research doing mining on distributed storage, using highly advanced new text, image and structured data mining on individual patients as well as on populations.

New knowledge will be fed into a Medical Knowledge Repository (MKR) and mixed with domain knowledge coming from external sources (guidelines and scientific evidence). Innovative and user friendly knowledge representation paradigms will be developed in order to enable not only knowledge engineers but also clinicians to use the repository

After validating, this knowledge will be used by a decision support module (DSM) and monitoring tool in the clinical environment to prevent patient safety issues and report on them, both at the population and at the patient level for direct care.

Co-ordination and steering of both the analysis and the care process will be done by a performant and versatile reasoning engine.

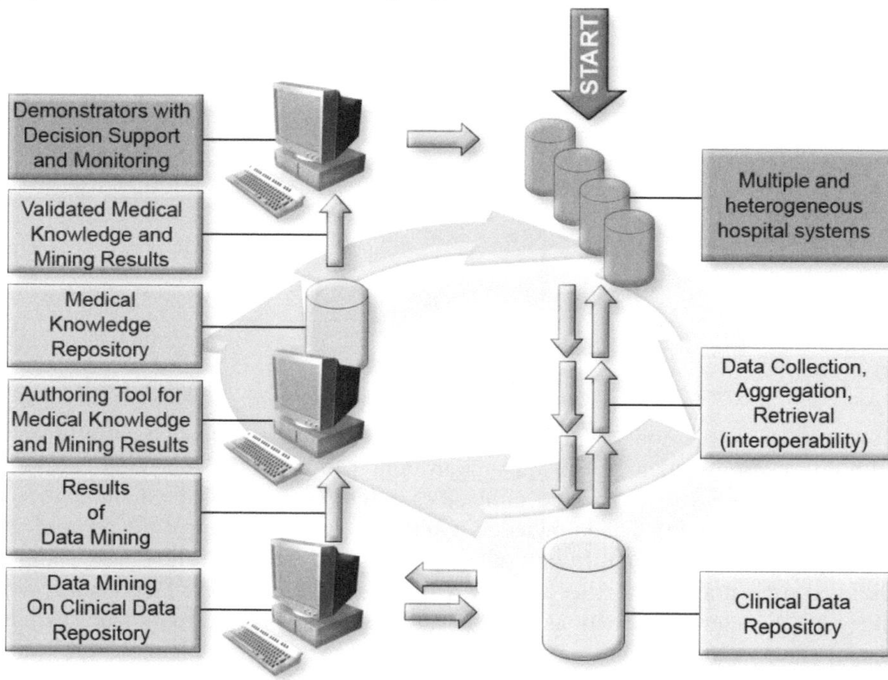

Figure 2: Overview of the project

4. Data Integration Approaches

There are currently a few different approaches proposed to integrate distributed heterogeneous data sources: link integration, data warehousing, view integration, workflows, and mashups.

According to their architectural model, these approaches can be classified either as centralised or decentralised. Another way to characterize them uses data overlapping. Where there is no data overlapping across the sources they can then be viewed as horizontal and, in the opposite case as vertical. Finally, for any integration approach, the access to the data can be via a push mechanism, where data is pushed into a periodically materialised database, or by a pull method, when a view on data is provided on demand.

a) Data warehousing

Data warehousing is a centralised approach that stores all the data of the sharing sites into one central database. In this approach, a unified data model is defined in order to accommodate all the information contained in the source sites. In addition, wrappers are created for each participant site in order to upload and manage the local data, so that it fits into the central database schema. Then, all the queries can be easily submitted centrally. Some projects using this approach are the Genome Database (IGD) project, ATLAS, BioWarehouse, and BioDWH.

High performance can be considered as one of the highest advantages of this system. In addition, it allows the user to modify and annotate the data since this is a replica, not the production database. There exist also other well-known techniques to build dynamic and online data navigation (OLAP) functionalities upon data warehouses that could serve the users for their data analyses.

This well-known industrial approach to data integration has proven to be efficient for relatively simple industrial contexts. In life science, with its fast evolving knowledge domain as well as the complexity of domain data models, this approach is less widely used due to the cost of data model updates in the central data stores, and to the additional risk of data exposure it leads to.

b) View Integration

View integration is a decentralised approach where source data is kept only in the source site. A single view around all the databases that share information within the system is created. Queries are converted into a common query language that is later handled by a mediator. The mediator identifies the sources that need to be accessed to retrieve the result. Then, it splits the query in many sub queries that are passed to wrappers. Those will transform their sub queries into the local language using mapping rules metadata, and access the data. After the data is fetched from the different sources, the result is globally integrated and returned to the user. HEMSYS [8] and TAMBIS [9] are examples of systems that follow this approach. Ontologies are usually used for view integration to help in aligning different data sources into a global concept of the data. The system can use either integration with a global ontology as in SIMS [10], where each source references the same domain ontology; or local ontology as in KRAFT [11].

When view integration is used, the data is always up to date and there is a relative decoupling from the data sources to the integration system. In the downside, usually the performance is not good since the loading of the data is on-demand and relies on the underlying network performance.

c) Others approaches

In the link integration approach, entries in a data source, usually a web page, are linked to other entries in another data sources via the integration system. SRS, one of the most used integration systems, follows this approach. Entrez and Integr8 are other examples.

Mashups are a Web 2.0 idea beginning to take hold in the life sciences. Mashups provide means to take data from more than one web-based resource and make a new web application. An example is the use of Google Earth to track the global spread of avian flu. Mashup development framework such as Google Mashup Editor, Microsoft's Popfly and Yahoo! Pipes speed up the development of mashups.

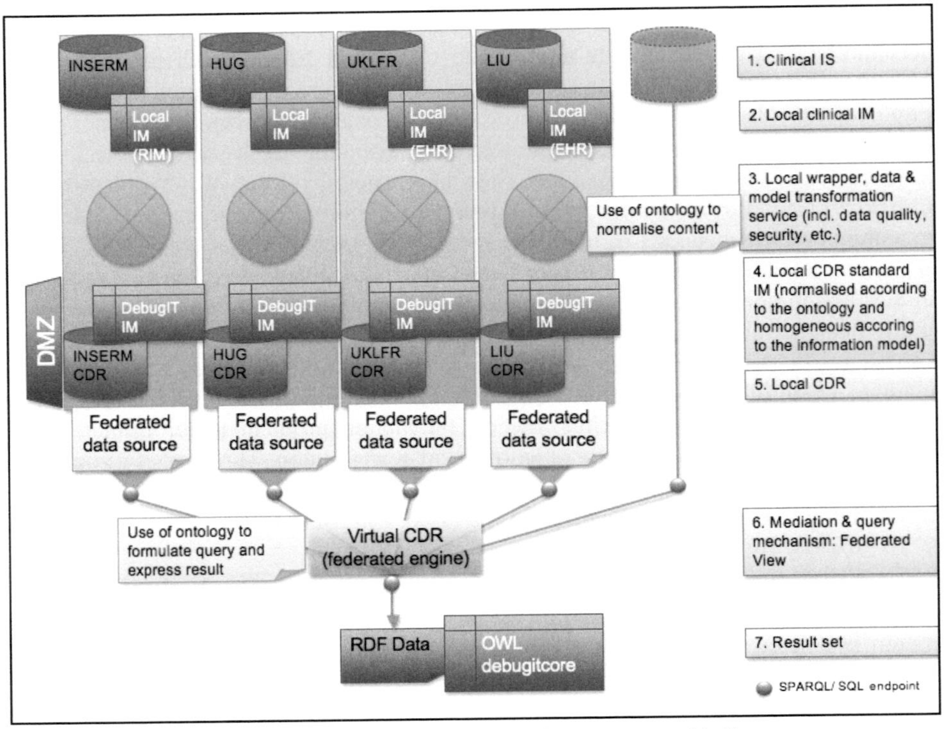

Figure 3. DebugIT CDR architecture. (acronyms: see table 1)

5. Dealing With Rules, Information and Knowledge

Another very important challenge is the ability to formalize existing rules, guidelines and other types of medical knowledge within a knowledge repository, which will hold new acquired knowledge. A very short example is given hereafter. Manually-generated rules are based on clinical guidelines provided by healthcare institutions. Typical recommendations are useful to prescribe the most appropriate antibiotic, according to different parameters, such as costs, benefits, adverse effects, as well as the risk of resistance development. As case study, we started investigating guidelines for the geriatrics (cf. Table 1) and the surgery services from the University Hospitals of Geneva (HUG).

Table 2. Slightly simplified sample of the guidelines

Pathologies	Pathogenic agents	Antibiotics	Alternatives	Treatment duration
Cholecystitis	Enterobacteriaceae Enterococcus Clostridium sp	ceftriaxone 1 g/24h iv + metronidazole 500 mg/8h iv	amoxi./clav. 1,2 g/8h iv	10-14 days
Gastroenteritis	Campylobacter Salmonella E. Coli Shigella (rare)	ciprofloxacine 500 mg/12h po	co-trimoxazole forte (160mg TMP/ 800mg SMX)/12h po & clarithromycine 500 mg/12h po	5-10 days

To transform such verbose documents into machine-readable data, the guidelines are transformed into databases tuples. The translation from French to English was performed manually, assisted by French-to-English translation tools (e.g. http://eagl.unige.ch/EAGLm/), and a SNOMED categorizer [6]. For some of the queries, several answers were possible – three on average – as shown in Table 2, where *diverticulitis* caused by *enterococcus* can be treated by three different antibiotics: *Ceftriaxone*, *Metronidazole* and *Piperacillin-Tazobactam*; each of them is unambiguously associated to a unique terminological identifier.

Automatically-generated rules are represented as triplets: 1) disease, 2) pathogen and 3) antibiotic. The objective of the automatic rule generation is to generate one of the items (so-called the *target*) of the triplet using the other two items (so-called the *sources*). The discovery of the third item relies on an advanced question-answering engine (EAGLi: Engine for Question Answering in Genomic Literature, http://eagl.unige.ch/EAGLi). Thus, the rule induction problem is reformulated as a question-answering problem, with a unique semantic solution. Three types of questions are designed:

1. Drug: Which *antibiotic* should be used against *this pathogen* causing *this disease*?
2. Pathogen: Which *pathogen* is responsible for *this disease* treated by *this antibiotic*?
3. Disease: Which *disease* is caused by *this pathogen* and treated by *this antibiotic*?

Further, two search engines, corresponding to different search models were tested: easyIR (a relevance-driven search engine well known for outperforming other search methods on MEDLINE search tasks [7] and PubMed (the NCBI's Boolean search instrument). All targets were normalized using standard terminologies: antibiotics and diseases in SNOMED CT or MeSH and bacteria in NEWT. To find the antibiotics, given disease and its pathogen, a list of 72 antibiotic targets was defined, corresponding mostly to the UMLS Semantic Type T195. To find the bacterial pathogens, given the disease and the antibiotic, we suggested a subset of the NEWT terminology corresponding to the bacteria taxonomy. To find pathological processes, knowing the pathogen and the antibiotic, we proposed a list of MeSH terms corresponding to disease, corresponding to the following UMLS Semantic Types T020|T190|T049|T019|T047|T050|T033|T037|T047|T191|T046|T184. For the antibiotics category, we tested the use of both SNOMED CT and the MeSH. Synonyms from these terminologies were also evaluated. Thus, "amoxycillin with clavulanate potassium" can also be mentioned as "amoxicillin-clavulanic acid" or "augmentin".

Furthermore, tuning the question-answering module includes terminology pruning. Indeed, several descriptors, in particular generic ones, need to be removed. Thus, *infectious diseases* or *cross-infection* were removed from the descriptor list for the disease type of target. Finally, specific keywords were used to refine the search equation in order to retrieve more accurate results. Thus, we added context specific descriptors such as *geriatrics*, *elderly*, for geriatric guidelines, etc. The impact of general keywords was also tested such as *recommended antibiotic*, *antibiotherapy*, etc.

6. Privacy

Strong attention is given to privacy concerns, taking into account the various legal and ethical frameworks to be met. Therefore, privacy is made a central part of the project *by design,* using a virtualized data repository without dealing directly with the original data. Identification elements provided by the clinical data repositories can be carried all along the process, blindly, in order to allow the original clinical information system to feed back decision support without need for patient identification.

7. Conclusion

The DebugIT project is focused on using large existing and heterogeneous clinical datasets covering hundreds of thousands of patients from several clinical information systems in different European countries. DebugIt proposes to build an interoperability platform to populate a pertinent dataset about the infectious domain to achieve a very large common shared virtualized clinical repository that enables knowledge-driven data mining. This "semantic mining" will be based on innovative methodologies to deal with the characteristics of real world clinical data. A knowledge repository will drive the data mining and serve as storehouse for the results. Finally, a decision support engine will exploit the aggregated knowledge to loop-back to the real world.

To achieve this system, several aspects will have to reach the frontiers of current state-of-the-art and beyond. Two strategies can be chosen for that. The first one is to invent something radically new. The second one consists of using all existing knowledge and methods, putting them together, and trying to build upon this base. For most of its research, the second strategy is the one chosen in this project, because operational results for clinical information systems must be available and sustain the DebugIT outcomes after the end of the project.

In order to meet these requirements, the project has been organized according to architectural component-based considerations:

- Interoperability Platform (IOP);
- Clinical Data Repository (CDR);
- Multimodal Data Mining (MDM);
- Medical Knowledge Repository and associated Knowledge Authoring Tool (MDR)
- Decision Support and Monitoring engine (DSM);
- Clinical applications.

This scientific and technical framework, associated with access to large amounts of clinical databases and led by experts in the medical field will lead to a serious advance in building a large IT infrastructure aiming at creating new knowledge in the field of monitoring, surveillance and efficient measures to fight infectious diseases.

References

[1] IOM. The computer-based Patient record: An essential technology for health care. Institute of Medicine report. 1991, revised 1997.

[2] Medicine Io, editor. To Err is Human. Building a safer Health System; 1999. National Academy Press.

[3] Frazee BW. Update on emerging infections: news from the Centers for Disease Control and Prevention. Severe methicillin-resistant Staphylococcus aureus community-acquired pneumonia associated with influenza--Louisiana and Georgia, December 2006-January 2007. Ann Emerg Med. 2007 Nov;50(5):612-6.
[4] O'Brien J A, Lahue BJ, Caro JJ, Davidson DM. The Emerging Infectious Challenge of Clostridium difficile-Associated Disease in Massachusetts Hospitals: Clinical and Economic Consequences. Infect Control Hosp Epidemiol. 2007 Nov;28(11):1219-27.
[5] McAlonan GM, Lee AM, Cheung V, Cheung C, Tsang KW, Sham PC, et al. Immediate and sustained psychological impact of an emerging infectious disease outbreak on health care workers. Canadian journal of psychiatry. 2007 Apr;52(4):241-7.
[6] Ruch P, Gobeill J, Lovis C, Geissbuhler A. Automatic medical encoding with SNOMED categories. BMC Med Inform Decis Mak. 2008;8 Suppl 1:S6.
[7] Aronson A DD-FD, Humphrey S, Lin J, Liu H, Ruch P, Ruiz M, Smith L, Tanabe L, Wilbur J. Fusion of knowledge-intensive and statistical approaches for retrieving and annotating textual genomics documents TREC National Institute of Standards and Technology. 2005.
[8] S. V. Pillai, R. Gudipati and L. Lilien, Design issues and an architecture for a heterogenous multidatabase system. Proceedings of the 15th ACM Computer Science Conference (1987).
[9] C. A. Goble et al., Transparent access to multiple bioinformatics information sources. IBM SYSTEMS JOURNAL 40 (2001), 532-551.
[10] The SIMS Corpus Project: http://groups.ischool.berkeley.edu/SIMSCorpus/results.htm
[11] A. D. Preece et al., The KRAFT Architecture for Knowledge Fusion and Transformation. Proceedings of the 19th SGES Int. Conf. on Knowledge-based Systems and Applied Artificial Intelligence (1999).

Part B

Detection and Prevention of Adverse Drug Events

Detection and Prevention of Adverse Drug Events
R. Beuscart et al. (Eds.)
IOS Press, 2009

doi:10.3233/978-1-60750-043-8-63

Detection of Adverse Drug Events: Proposal of a Data Model

Emmanuel CHAZARD[a, 1], Béatrice MERLIN[a], Grégoire FICHEUR[a], Jean-Charles SARFATI[b], the PSIP Consortium and Régis BEUSCART[a]
[a]*Lille university hospital, EA2694, France*
[b]*Oracle France SAS*

Abstract. Our main objective is to detect adverse drug events (ADEs) in former hospital stays. As ADEs are rare, that supposes to screen thousands of electronic health records (EHRs). For that purpose, we need to define a data model that has two main objectives: (1) being able to describe hospital stays from various hospitals (2) being tuned so as to prepare the data mining process: as ADEs are not flagged in the datasets, the data model must be optimized for ADE detection. The article presents the phases of the design and the data model that results from this work. It is compatible with many hospitals. It deals with diagnoses, drug prescriptions, lab results and administrative information. It allows for data mining and ADE detection in EHRs.

Keywords. Adverse drug event detection, data-mining, data model, interoperability.

Introduction

Adverse drug events (ADEs) are a public health issue. Usually, they are detected thanks to non automated methods that encounter several issues:

- Time consuming staff operated reviews: but as ADEs are rare events, the probability of a case to be observed remains low.
- Spontaneous ADE declarations: most often physicians only declare ADEs that are rare or severe and do not result from a reprehensible fault. As a consequence, those declarations only report a low proportion of ADEs [1, 2].

So there is a need for automated ADE detection methods that could allow for large datasets screening. Electronic Health Records (EHRs) are considered to be very useful in the field of ADEs [3, 4] because big amounts of data are routinely collected and allow for a wide retrospective analysis. The objective of our project is to use data mining methods such as decision trees [5-10] and association rules [11, 12] to automatically identify ADEs from EHRs from several French and Danish hospitals. This will help to automatically discover some prevention rules. After a validation step those rules will be implemented into a Clinical decision support system (CDSS).

The first step of that project is to propose a common data model and to feed it with data in respect with the model. In this article we will present the approach we use and

[1] Corresponding Author: Dr Emmanuel Chazard, CHRU de Lille, 2 avenue Oscar Lambret, 59000 Lille, France; E-mail: emmanuel@chazard.org.

the data model we obtain. In our approach, the data model is considered as a strong link in the chain:

- Upstream, the data model has to be compliant with all the available data from French and Danish partners
- Downstream, the data model has to be tuned in order to allow data mining to detect ADEs although they are not explicitly flagged in the data: no field tells "ADE: yes/no". If such a field was available, it wouldn't be reliable.

1. Material and Methods

1.1. Review of Cases

Our aim is to formalize experts' decision process: assuming a patient encountered an ADE, what part of the available data helped the experts' advice? A record review is first performed. 90 atypical hospital stays are reviewed by physicians assisted by a computer scientist.

They are asked to answer the following questions:

- *Was there a probable ADE?*
- *If yes, how did you notice there was an ADE?*
- *Is it possible to generalize those criteria as a rule; would new aggregated fields be useful to that?*
- *Does this case inspire you other detectable situations?*

As an example, two clinical cases of ADEs, and the corresponding variables are presented in Table 1 & Table 2. This procedure is followed up and generalized on every available fields (Table 3).

Table 1. First example of ADE case and inferred variable

Clinical case (ADE)	Mr. X had been admitted for phlebitis, treated and discharged. The treatment wasn't well adapted. The patient bled and had to come back two days later.
What abnormality is visible in the EHR?	The patient had to come back 2 days later
What variable(s) could be useful?	*dunh*=delay up to next hospitalization. In present case *dunh*=2.
Examples of possible uses of the new variable(s)	Binary use: ifelse(*dunh*< arbitrary_threshold; 1; 0) ifelse(*dunh*< defined_quantile; 1; 0) Quantitative use: 1/(*dunh*+1) *equals 0 if the patient never comes back*

Table 2. Second example of ADE case and inferred variable

Clinical case (ADE)		Mr. Y had been admitted in relation with appendicitis and died 4 days later from grand mal status epilepticus.
Abnormality #1	**What abnormality is visible in the EHR?**	The patient had been admitted for appendicitis but died
	What variable(s) could be useful?	*Death* {0;1}, in present case *Death*=1. *DRG** $\{d_1; d_2;\ldots; d_k\}$, in present case *DRG*=d_i. Expected death knowing the DGR = *exp_death*= P(*Death*| *DRG*=d_i)

	Examples of possible uses of the new variable(s)	Binary use: *death* ifelse(*exp_death*<0.05 & *death*=1; 1; 0) Quantitative use: ifelse(*death*=1; log(*exp_death*); 0) ifelse(*death*=1; log(*exp_death*); log(1-*exp_death*))
Abnorm. #2	**What abnormality is visible in the EHR?**	Principal diagnosis of first step of the hospital stay is appendicitis and principal diagnosis of the second step of the stay is epilepsy: those diagnoses concern two different medical specialties.
	What variable(s) could be useful?	Theoretical MDC* of the principal diagnosis of each step *ntmdc*= Number of different theoretical MDCs in the whole stay in present case *ntmdc*=2
	Examples of possible uses of the new variable(s)	Binary use: ifelse(*ntmdc*>1; 1; 0) Quantitative use: *ntmdc* - 1

* DRG: diagnosis related group MDC: major disease category (group of DRGs, medical specialty)

Table 3. Examples of fields' exploitation (ideas)

Native variable	**Idea of use**	**Maybe useful as…**
Death	Unlikelihood of the death	ADE detection
ZIP code	Distance from home to the hospital Does the patient live in the region? Does the patient live in urban area?	potential cause potential cause potential cause
Gender	Usable as it	potential cause
External moves	Admittance day of week Entry by emergency Transfer to another hospital (acute care only)	potential cause potential cause ADE detection
Internal moves	Going through ICU* Back-and-forth patterns	ADE detection / potential cause ADE detection
Dates	Age Unexpected high length of stay Short delay up to next hospitalization	potential cause ADE detection ADE detection
Diagnosis	Chronic diseases, admittance grounds ADE-related diagnosis codes Number of different theoretical MDCs*	potential cause ADE detection ADE detection
Lab result	Pre-existing abnormality Abnormality occurring during the hospital stay	potential cause ADE detection
Drug	Drug prescriptions Specific antidotes, some unexpected prescriptions	potential cause ADE detection

* ICU: intensive care unit MDC: major disease category (group of DRGs, medical specialty)

1.2. Review of the Available Data, Cardinalities and Encoding Systems

A review of the available data is performed to answer the following questions:

- What structured data are available in each partner's EHR?

- What part of those data is mandatory in all the country due to the administrative payment system?
- What part of those data should be available since it is the simplest way to describe information?
- What part of the data could be unreliable or unstable over time?

Then a review of data schemes and cardinality is performed:

- What would be the simplest way to store lab results / drug prescriptions / diagnoses / administrative information?
- Are the available data schemes of the partners able to feed such a relational scheme?

Finally a review of encoding systems allows us to choose common classifications.

1.3. Compromise

We have to reach a compromise from all those considerations in order to define the data scheme. That compromise is reached together by physicians, medical informatics scientists and statisticians over two main axes:

- cardinality of the scheme (number of tables):
  - o less relationships: easier data quality control, easier data mining by statisticians
  - o more relationships: data closer from the native scheme, easier extraction, less errors, more stability over time
- number of columns (fields):
  - o more columns: more data provisions and calculated fields
  - o less columns: faster extraction, less errors, compatibility over countries and time

2. Results

2.1. Encoding Systems

Diagnoses are encoded using the ICD10 classification [13] (International statistical Classification of Diseases and related health problems, 10th Revision) of the World Health Organization.

DRGs are encoded using the national classifications (French or Danish). The choice of the classification does not have any impact since the groups are only used to compute aggregated statistics that are used in their turn instead of the DRG itself: death frequency, average length of stay, ICU frequency…

Drugs are encoded using the ATC classification [14] (Anatomical and Therapeutic Classification). That classification is not the most precise one but its precision was sufficient for statistical analysis. Moreover it is widely used.

Lab results are encoded using the C-NPU classification (Commission on Nomenclature Properties and Units) of the International Union of Pure and Applied Chemistry [15]. That classification is used by our partners and is chosen because of its ability to take into account units at the opposite of other popular classifications. That point is mandatory to detect abnormal values.

Medical procedures are encoded using local French or Danish classifications. It is not possible to enforce a common system. However the limited uses allows considering partial handmade mappings.

2.2. Data Scheme Presentation

Figure 1 shows a simplified representation of the data scheme, on which fields are replaced with groups of fields. The data scheme is voluntary not completely normalized as the data are updated from clean transactional databases and are never modified in the repository itself.

Medical and administrative information: the "1- Stays" table contains one row per hospitalization stay. One stay can be made up of one to several steps (emergency, ICU, cardiology…). The "2- Steps of the stay" table contains one row per step. Diagnoses and medical procedures are linked to the steps of the hospital stays.

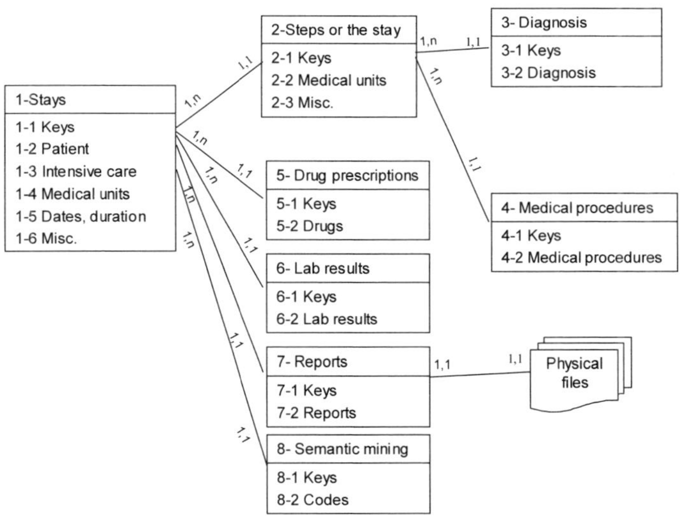

Figure 1. Simplified representation of the data scheme

Drug prescriptions: data-mining is performed stay per stay and details under the day level will be ignored. For a given hospital stay, drug prescriptions must be summed day per day in respect with the administered drug. Drugs corresponding to several ATC codes should be duplicated. Formally speaking, the doses of the drugs are summed and grouped by the {id_hospital, id_stay, date, drug_name, ATC_code} unique quintuplet.

Lab results: one row of the table corresponds to one assessment of one parameter at a given time. If available, each record should contain the normality range (bounds).

Free text data: every report is stored as a physical file linked to its hospital stay thanks to a specific table. Some of our partners use semantic mining to generate ICD10 and ATC codes from reports. A specific table allows registering those codes.

The required data do not contain any nominative nor indirectly nominative data such as birth date, ZIP code or exact dates.

2.3. Fields Detailed Description

The data scheme contains 8 tables from which 2 are dedicated to reports and 89 fields from which 60 are not identifiers. The field list is shown in Table 4 **Table 5** Table 6 Table 7 Table 8 Table 9 Table 10 & Table **11**. The original version of the scheme description is completed by detailed description of each field. It is not possible to print it here. That scheme is completed by physical files for the reports.

Table 4. The hospital stay table

Group	Field	Field (long name)	origin	unit
Keys	id_hosp	Hospital ID number	constant	ID number
	id_stay	Stay ID number	database	ID number
	id_patient	Patient ID number	database	ID number
	id_stay_mother	if it was a childbirth, the ID of the mother's stay	database	ID number
	id_stay_newborn	if it was a delivery (childbirth), the ID of the newborn's stay	database	ID number
Patient	age	Age	database	years (float)
	gender	Gender	database	0/1
	drg	Diagnosis Related Group	database	DRG code
	death_01	Death during the stay	database	0/1
	death_exp	Expected frequency of death in this DRG	the proportion in the whole hospital for each DRG	proportion, float between 0 and 1
	geo_state_01	Does the patient come from the hospital's country (state)?	constant	0/1
	geo_region_01	Does the patient come from the hospital's region?	geographic reference	0/1
	geo_dpt_01	Does the patient come from the hospital's department?	geographic reference	0/1
	p_diag	Principal diagnosis	database	ICD10 code
	drg_eff	Number of stays used to compute the various DRG-based statistics (duration_exp, deth_exp, duration_icu_exp, throught_icu_exp)	the number of stays computed in the whole hospital for this DRG	integer
ICU	through_icu_01	Taken care of in intensive care/resuscitation unit?	database	0/1
	through_icu_exp	Expected frequency of stays with intensive care/resuscitation for this DRG	the proportion computed in the whole hospital for each DRG	proportion, float between 0 and 1

	duration_icu	Duration in an intensive care/resuscitation unit	database	days (integer)
	duration_icu_exp	Expected duration in an intensive care/resuscitation unit	the average duration computed in the whole hospital for each DRG	days (float)
	saps	Gravity score	database	integer
	duration_icu_sd	Standard deviation of the duration in an intensive care/resuscitation unit	the std dev of the duration computed in the whole hospital for each DRG	days (float)
	delay_icu	Delay before ICU/resuscitation step	database	integer
Places	nb_mu	Number of medical units visited during the stay	database	integer
	back_forth_01	Back and forth between medical units	database	0/1
	from_emergency_01	Was the patient admitted by an emergency unit?	database	0/1
Dates	duration	Duration of the stay	database	days (integer)
	duration_exp	Expected duration for the stays of this DRG	the average duration computed in the whole hospital for this DRG	days (float)
	delay_next_hosp	Delay up to next hospitalization	database	days (integer)
	duration_sd	Standard deviation of the duration for the stays of this DRG	the std dev of the duration computed in the whole hospital for this DRG	days (float)
Misc	nb_th_mdc	Number of different theoretical MDCs (Major Diagnostic Categories)	table "steps of the stay"	integer
	transfer_entry_01	Transfer from another hospital (whatever the kind)	database	0/1
	transfer_01	Transfer to another acute care hospital	database	0/1
	nb_proc	Number of different medical procedures	database	integer
	nb_diags	Number of different associated diagnosis	database	integer
	weight	weight of the patient	database	float

Table 5. The steps of the hospital stays table

Group	Field	Field (long name)	origin	unit
Keys	id_hosp	Hospital ID number	constant	ID number
	id_stay	Stay ID number	database	ID number
	id_step_stay	StayStep ID number	database	ID number
	id_patient	Patient ID number	database	ID number
Places	mu	Medical unit of the step	database	name
	icu_01	Is it an intensive care unit?	database	0/1
	emergency_01	Is it an emergency room?	database	0/1
Misc	saps	Gravity score	database	integer
	p_diag	Principal diagnosis of step of the stay	database	ICD10 code
	th_mdc	Theoretical MDC of the principal diagnosis	external ICD related table	integer
	weight	weight of the patient during the step	database	float
	step_stay_rank	the rank of that step in the stay (1 for the first step, 2 for the second one, …, k)	database	integer
	duration	Duration of the step of the stay	database	days (integer)

Table 6. The diagnoses table

Group	Field	Field (long name)	origin	unit
Keys	id_hosp	Hospital ID number	constant	name
	id_stay	Stay ID number	database	ID number
	id_step_stay	StayStep ID number	database	ID number
	id_patient	Patient ID number	database	ID number
Diagnosis	diag	Associated diagnosis	database	ICD10 code

Table 7. The medical procedures table

Group	Field	Field (long name)	origin	unit
Keys	id_hosp	Hospital ID number	constant	ID number
	id_stay	Stay ID number	database	ID number
	id_step_stay	StayStep ID number	database	ID number
	id_patient	Patient ID number	database	ID number
Procedures	proc	Medical procedure	database	act code
	delay_proc	delay between the entry and the procedure execution	database	Days (integer)

Table 8. The drug table

Group	Field	Field (long name)	origin	unit
Keys	id_hosp	Hospital ID number	constant	ID number
	id_stay	Stay ID number	database	ID number
	id_patient	Patient ID number	database	ID number
Drugs	name	Commercial name	database	name
	atc	ATC Code	external drugs related table	name
	delay_drug	delay between the entry and the administration	database	Days (integer)
	dose	total drug dose administered during this day	database	number
	unit	Unit used for the total dose	database	name
	route	Route	database	name

Table 9. The lab results table

Group	Field	Field (long name)	origin	unit
Keys	id_hosp	Hospital ID number	constant	ID number
	id_stay	Stay ID number	database	ID number
	id_patient	Patient ID number	database	ID number
Lab	delay_bio	delay between the entry and the sample	database	Days (integer)
	cnpu	C-NPU identifier (IUPAC) of the setting (NPU01685…)	database or external joint	string
	value	value	database	float
	unit	unit used for the value	database	string
	up_bound	upper bound	database	float
	lo_bound	lower bound	database	float

Table 10. The reports table

Group	Field	Field (long name)	origin	unit
Keys	id_hosp	Hospital ID number	constant	ID number
	id_stay	Stay ID number	database	ID number
	id_patient	Patient ID number	database	ID number
Reports	kind	kind of text	database	String
	filename	filename	database	String

Table 11. The semantic mining table

Group	Field	Field (long name)	origin	unit
Keys	id_hosp	Hospital ID number	constant	ID number
	id_stay	Stay ID number	database	ID number
	id_patient	Patient ID number	database	ID number
Codes	terminology	Terminology or nomenclature name	external terminologies	String
	kind	kind of text	database	String
	code	Code of the term	external database	String
	term	Name of the term	external database	String

2.4. Extraction Process

Data extraction has been developed in each hospital. A local mechanism is in charge of extracting data directly into tabulated text files. As the same format is used by the statistical software, there is no need for database loading before the data mining process. Nevertheless, a database is used for other needs (Figure 2).

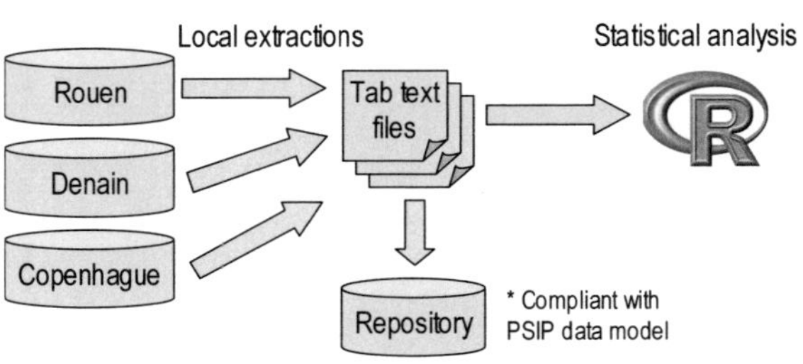

Figure 2. Current data extraction

3. Conclusion

3.1. Perspectives

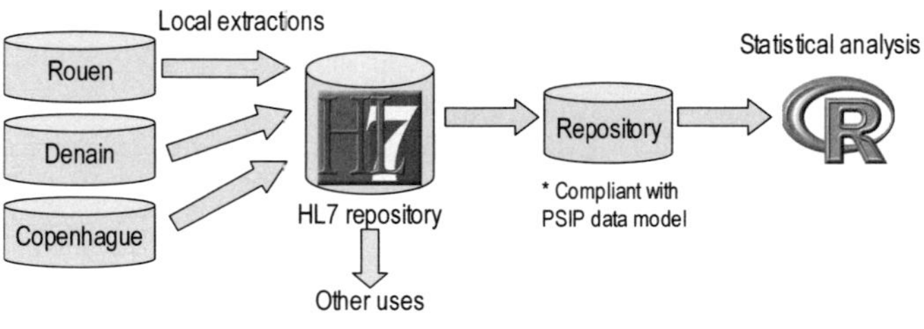

Figure 3. Future data extraction

In the future a central database will be used. That repository will implement an HL7 [16] compatible data scheme. Downstream our data model will still be used to feed the data mining step. The use of HL7 won't improve the process itself but will be useful when new partners join the project. Hospitals that are already able to extract data according to HL7 standards will feed our repository much faster (Figure 3).

3.2. Other Uses

The data model has already shown its relevancy since the extraction could be quickly performed and the data mining could be processed and generate interesting results [17]. Moreover, this data model is currently being adapted to another European project. As the study won't concern anymore hospitalizations but long-term follows-up, the data model has to be complemented in order to incorporate more patient-related data and ambulatory care related data.

Acknowledgement

The research leading to these results has received funding from the European Community's Seventh Framework Program (FP7/2007-2013) [18, 19] under Grant Agreement n° 216130 - the PSIP project [20].

References

[1] Morimoto T, Gandhi TK, Seger AC, Hsieh TC, Bates DW. Adverse drug events and medication errors: detection and classification methods. Qual Saf Health Care. 2004 Aug;13(4):306-14.
[2] Murff HJ, Patel VL, Hripcsak G, Bates DW. Detecting adverse events for patient safety research: a review of current methodologies. J Biomed Inform. 2003 Feb-Apr;36(1-2):131-43.
[3] Gurwitz JH, Field TS, Harrold LR, Rothschild J, Debellis K, Seger AC, et al. Incidence and preventability of adverse drug events among older persons in the ambulatory setting. JAMA. 2003 Mar 5;289(9):1107-16.
[4] Jalloh OB, Waitman LR. Improving Computerized Provider Order Entry (CPOE) usability by data mining users' queries from access logs. AMIA Annu Symp Proc. 2006:379-83.
[5] Zhang HP, Crowley J, Sox H, Olshen RA. Tree structural statistical methods. Encyclopedia of Biostatistics. Chichester, England: Wiley; 2001. p. 4561-73.
[6] Breiman L. Classification and regression trees. Belmont, Calif.: Wadsworth International Group; 1984.
[7] Fayyad U, Piatetsky-Shapiro G, Smyth P, editors. From data mining to knowledge discovery : an overview. 2nd Int Conf on Knowledge Discovery and Data Mining; 1996.
[8] Lavrac N. Selected techniques for data mining in medicine. Artif Intell Med. 1999 May;16(1):3-23.
[9] Quinlan JR. Introduction of Decision Trees. Machine Learning. 1986;1:81-106.
[10] Ripley BD. Pattern recognition and neural networks. Cambridge ; New York: Cambridge University Press; 1996.
[11] Agrawal R, Imielinski T, Swami A, editors. Mining Association Rules between Sets of Items in Large Databases. Proceedings of the ACM SIGMOD International Conference on Management of Data; 1993 May. Washington D.C.
[12] Piatetsky-Shapiro G, Frawley W. Knowledge discovery in databases. Menlo Park, Calif.: AAAI Press : MIT Press; 1991.

[13] International Classification of Diseases. [cited 2009 february 24]; Available from: http://www.who.int/classifications/icd/en.
[14] Anatomical and Therapeutical Classification. [cited 2009 february 24]; Available from: http://www.whocc.no/atcddd.
[15] International Union of Pure and Applied Chemistry. [cited 2009 february 24]; Available from: http://www.iupac.org.
[16] Health level 7. [cited 2009 April 21]; Available from: http://www.hl7.org/.
[17] Chazard E, Preda C, Merlin B, Ficheur G, Beuscart R. Data-mining-based detection of adverse drug events. Stud Health Technol Inform. 2009;[IN PRESS].
[18] European Research Council. [cited 2009 february 24]; Available from: http://erc.europa.eu.
[19] Seventh Framework programme. [cited 2009 february 24]; Available from: http://cordis.europa.eu/fp7/home_en.html.
[20] Patient Safety by Intelligent Procedures in medication. [cited 2009 february 24]; Available from: http://www.psip-project.eu.

Detection and Prevention of Adverse Drug Events
R. Beuscart et al. (Eds.)
IOS Press, 2009

doi:10.3233/978-1-60750-043-8-75

Detection of Adverse Drug Events Detection: Data Agregation and Data Mining

Emmanuel CHAZARD [a, 1], Grégoire FICHEUR [a], Béatrice MERLIN [a], Michael GENIN[a], Cristian PREDA [b], the PSIP consortium and Régis BEUSCART [a]
[a] *Lille university hospital, EA2694, France*
[b] *Lille 1 sciences and technology university, France*

Abstract. Adverse drug events (ADEs) are a public health issue. The objective of this work is to data-mine electronic health records in order to automatically identify ADEs and generate alert rules to prevent those ADEs. The first step of data-mining is to transform native and complex data into a set of binary variables that can be used as causes and effects. The second step is to identify cause-to-effect relationships using statistical methods. After mining 10,500 hospitalizations from Denmark and France, we automatically obtain 250 rules, 75 have been validated till now. The article details the data aggregation and an example of decision tree that allows finding several rules in the field of vitamin K antagonists.

Keywords. Data mining, adverse drug events, decision trees, association rules, anti-coagulation, vitamin K antagonists, INR.

Introduction

Adverse Drug Events (ADEs) are a public health issue. In some hospitals drugs are prescribed using a computerized provider order entry (CPOE) in the frame of the medication use process. In this case it is possible to couple the CPOE with a clinical decision support system (CDSS). It should be then theoretically possible to prevent ADEs by adding some alert rules, such as “aspirin & vitamin K antagonist => increased risk of bleeding”.

But in usual approaches the alert rules are specified by experts. The knowledge that is used usually relies on 2 main sources:

- Academic knowledge: this knowledge mainly relies on summaries of product characteristics and ADE declarations... but ADE declarations are known to only report a tiny proportion of ADEs [1, 2], mostly rare or grave events where the physician’s responsibility is not involved.
- Staff operated reviews (record reviews, chart reviews): those methods can consider very complex situations mixing diseases, drug characteristics and human factors. But they are time-consuming, mostly because ADEs are rare events so their observation requires the review of many normal cases [2].

Those rules induce another underestimated problem: they are applied in the same way to the medical departments all over the countries although those medical

[1] Corresponding Author: Dr Emmanuel Chazard, CHRU Lille, 2 avenue Oscar Lambret, 59000 Lille, France; E-mail: emmanuel@chazard.org.

departments vary a lot on several aspects. As a consequence in those classic approaches the alerts are too numerous and of poor accuracy. The physicians often complain of over-alerting and their confidence in the system decreases to such an extent that some of them use to deactivate the CDSS.

The main objective or the PSIP project (Patient Safety through Intelligent Procedures in medication [3]) is to build a CDSS relying on automated rules generation, taking into account the context. The objectives of the present work are:

1. to perform a data aggregation: the aim of this step is to transform complex data into events that could be usable as "causes" and "effects". This step is very important because of the complexity of the available data (many codes, repeated assessments over time, cardinalities of the data scheme, etc.)
2. to automatically data-mine [4] those data in order:
   - to identify adverse drug events
   - to generate control rules to prevent those ADEs

Two important points must be emphasized:

1. The process has to be able to detect ADEs in routine datasets. In those datasets, the ADEs are not flagged..
2. All the process must be automated so that it could be easily performed on new datasets.

1. Material and Methods

1.1. Available Data

Electronic Health Records (EHRs) seem to be the best data source in the field of ADEs [5, 6]. For the project we have designed a data model and implemented it in a central repository. This data model contains 8 tables and 92 fields (Figure).

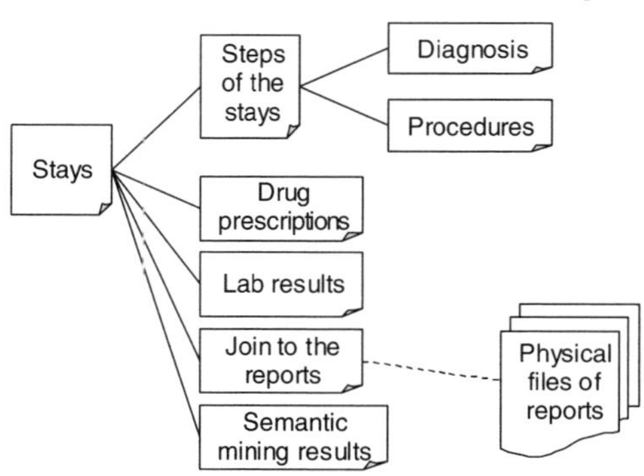

Figure 1. The 8 tables of the data model.

Data extractions are performed to feed the repository. An important point is that no data has to be specifically recorded for the project: we only use routinely collected data from EHRs. Those data include:

- medical and administrative information
- diagnosis encoded using ICD10 [7]
- medical procedures encoded using national classifications
- drug prescriptions encoded using the ATC classification [8]

- laboratory results encoded using the C-NPU classification (IUPAC) [9]

Data are extracted from EHRs provided by the hospitals involved in the project. An iterative quality control of the data is performed in order to get reliable data and to improve the extraction mechanisms. Data extraction is being continued, the present work is performed using 10,500 Danish and French hospital stays of year 2007, mostly from cardiologic or geriatric units:

- Capital Region of Denmark hospitals (Dk): 2,700 hospital stays
- Rouen university hospital (F): 800 hospital stays
- Denain hospital (F): 7,000 hospital stays

1.2. Our Hook to Fish ADEs

We follow a four-step procedure (Figure):

1. Transform the data into events: the native data are complex (thousands of codes, repeated assessments of various lab settings, etc.). They are transformed into binary events. Those events can happen or not. If they happen, they have a start date and a stop date.
2. Qualify the events as "potential cause of ADEs" or "potential effects of ADEs".
3. Automatically find statistical associations between causes and effects. At this step, associations do not necessary mean ADE. For instance we could find "age>90 & renal insufficiency => too long stay".
4. Filter the associations: associations that contain drugs in their list of causes are kept and are validated against academic knowledge.

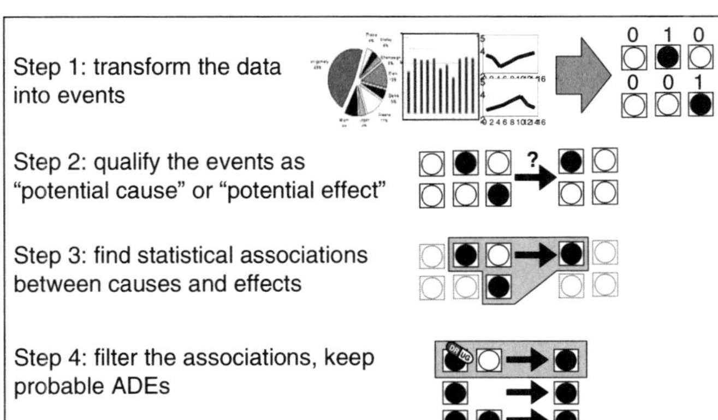

Figure 2. Our four-step procedure to fish ADEs.

1.3. Step 1: Transform the Data Into Event (Data Aggregation)

The extracted datasets fit an 8-tables relational scheme. But such a data repository cannot be used for statistical analysis:

- No statistical method can deal with an 8-tables data scheme
- The encoding systems allow for too numerous classes: about 17,000 codes for ICD10, about 5,400 codes for the ATC, and dozens of different settings for lab results. Many codes have comparable meanings (e.g. the concept of hypoxemia is accessible from the oxygen blood pressure or the oxygen

saturation of hemoglobin) and some concepts result from several settings (e.g. metabolic acidosis).
- Some variables have repeated assessments all the stay along, e.g. lab results (a red cells count can be assessed 20 times during the stay, returning normal, too low or too high values) or drug prescriptions (a specific drug can be prescribed twice per day), etc.

We develop aggregating engines to transform the available data into information described as sets of events (Figure 3). For each kind of data (administrative information, diagnoses, drugs, lab results), a specific aggregating engine is developed and fed with a specific aggregation policy. Each policy is described outside the engine, allowing for several persons to work in the same time to improve the aggregation phase. The aggregating engines allow getting a table that describes the events thanks to many binary fields.

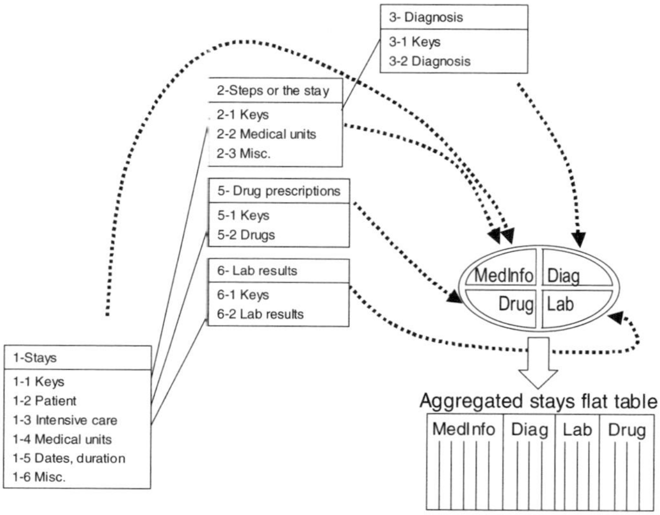

Figure 3. Aggregating engines and mapping policies

Classical statistical analyses rely on associations between different variables that are considered as *stable states*. This is true in some cases (e.g. a patient remains a man or a woman all the stay long) but most often it is false (e.g. a hypoalbuminemia, potential cause of some ADEs, might only exist at days 5, 6 & 7 of a 20-days-long stay). The engines transform data into events. For a given hospital stay, events can have one of the two values (Figure):
- 0: the event doesn't occur
- 1: the event occurs at least once. In that case, it is characterized by its start date and end date.

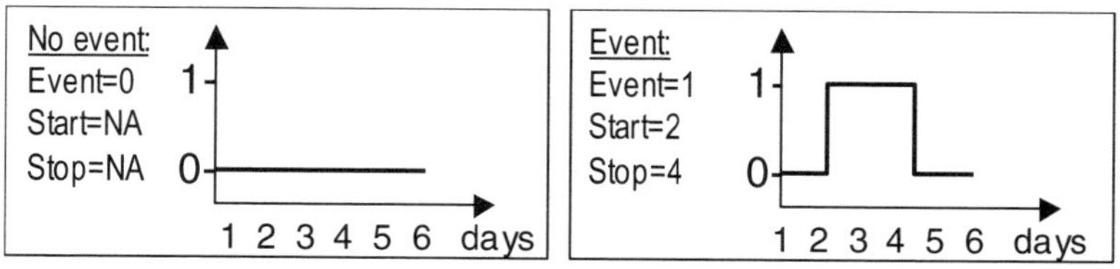

Figure 4. Events can be set to 0 or 1

Example of the Lab Results

As an example, let's examine the aggregation of the INR (international normalized ratio) values on one example of hospital stay. This setting is interesting for patients under vitamin K antagonists. The expected values are between 3 and 4.5. In this example, INR can assess 2 kinds of risky situations:

- When INR<3, the patient is exposed to a risk of thrombosis.
- When INR>4.5 the patient is exposed to a risk of bleeding.

The lab aggregating engine uses the lab mapping policies and is able to fill two binary variables: too_low_inr and too_high_inr. Those variables are accompanied by start dates and stop dates when their values are set to 1 (Figure). LOCF (last observation carried forward) is used to interpolate the available values.

Kind	Day offset	Value	Lower bound	Upper bound
INR	1	3.4	3	4.5
INR	3	3.2	3	4.5
INR	5	2.5	3	4.5
INR	8	2.9	3	4.5
INR	10	3.2	3	4.5
INR	15	3.6	3	4.5

Native data

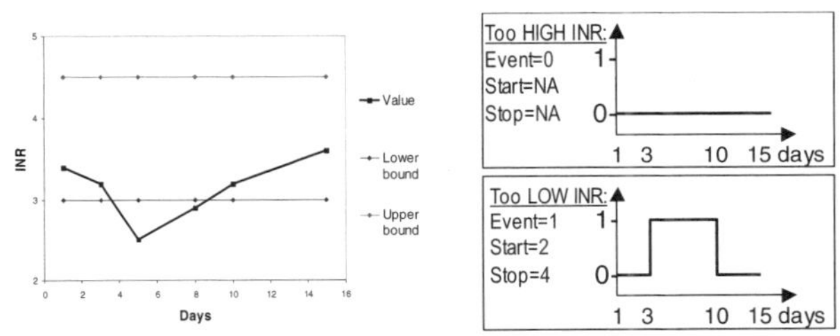

Chart of the values *2 binary variables & dates*

Figure 5. Example of transformation: the INR values of a stay

1.4. Step 2: Qualify the Events as "Potential Cause" or "Potential Effect"

We first perform an informal analysis: in the available data, some can be identified as "potential cause of an ADE" and some other as "potential effect of an ADE". Table shows examples of classifications.

Table 1. Examples of information classification: potential case / potential effect

Kind of information	Ex. of potential ADE cause	Ex. of potential ADE effect
Administrative information	Age, gender	Death, too long stay
Diagnosis	Chronic renal insufficiency	Hemorrhage at the middle of the stay
Lab results	Admission with a too high INR	Hyperkaliemia at the middle of the stay
Drug prescription	Vitamin K antagonist	Specific antidote

Finally thanks to the data-to-events transformation, it is possible to simply consider that all the events that occur after the patient's admittance are potential effects.

Example of the Lab Results

In this case (Figure), a too low INR occurred from the 3rd day (included) to the 10th day (excluded). Those two binary variables can be used as causes and as effects.

- too_low_inr (=1 from day 3 to day 9 in this case)
  - o is able to be an effect with value=1. All the other events that occur before day 3 will be candidate to explain that effect

  - o is able to be a cause for every effects that occur between day 3 and day 10
- too_high_inr (=0 all along in this case):
  - o is able to be an effect with value=0. All the other events will be candidate to explain the absence of effect, whatever their date
  - o is able to be a cause with value=0 for every effects, whenever they occur

This approach has two important advantages:

- A statistical association doesn't have any direction. But taking the dates into account prevents from causal relationship inversion. Events that are posterior to the effects cannot be interpreted as causes. Events that are anterior but too far from the effect are not taken into account.
- Effects can become causes in their turn. That approach allows considering an **ADE domino effect**. For instance:
  first drug A & age>70 => acute renal insufficiency
  then acute renal insufficiency & drug B => hemorrhage

1.5. Step 3: Automatically Find Statistical Associations Between Causes and Effects

The previous steps allow identifying potential ADE causes and potential ADE effects. The aim of statistical analysis is then to identify some links between (combination of) potential causes and potential effects. Decision trees [10-15] with the CART method were used thanks to the RPART package [16] of R [17]. Decision trees allow identifying several decision rules containing 1 to K conditions such as:

IF(condition_1 & … & condition_K) THEN outcome might occur

Each rule is characterized by its confidence (1: proportion of outcome knowing that the conditions are matched) and its support (2: proportion of records matching both conditions and outcome).

$$Confidence = P(\ outcome \mid condition\_1 \cap \ldots \cap condition\_K) \quad (1)$$

$$Support = P(\ outcome \cap condition\_1 \cap \ldots \cap condition\_K) \quad (2)$$

Rules are automatically produced.

1.6. Step 4: Filter the Associations, Keep Probable ADEs

The rules are then automatically filtered according to the following criteria:

- The rule must contain at least one of the following events type as a condition:
  - o one drug
  - o one drug suppression
  - o one lab result that is implicitly linked to a drug (e.g. INR for vitamin K antagonist, digoxinemia for digoxin…)
- The rule must increase the prevalence of the effect:
  Confidence > P(outcome)
- The rule must lead to a significant Fisher's exact test for independency between the set of conditions and the outcome.

A theoretical validation of the obtained rules is finally performed by physicians. Only rules that can be explained according to summaries of products characteristics and bibliography are kept. That review uses several drug-related web information portals [18-20], Pubmed [21] referenced papers, and French summaries of products characteristics provided by the Vidal company. In order to be sure the validated rules are reliable, the stays they allow to detect have to be reviewed by experts; this work is currently being processed.

2. Results

2.1. Data Aggregation

The figures that are presented here only reflect the current progress status, they are likely to change.

The 18,000 ICD10 codes are aggregated into 48 categories of chronic diseases.

The 5,400 ATC codes are aggregated into 242 drug categories. Those categories are designed to be redundant: they allow for transversal categories such as "hepatic enzyme inhibitors". The classification has to consider pharmacodynamics and pharmacokinetics although most of the existing classifications are based on therapeutic indications. Drug suppression is also traced as a potential ADE cause.

The laboratory results are aggregated into 35 lab abnormalities.

The various administrative fields are aggregated into 15 different variables.

The data aggregation produces one dataset per medical department. In each dataset up to 538 cause variables can be used to explain or predict 79 effect variables.

2.2. Decision Rules

Decision trees are systematically computed in order to explain each effect by all the available potential causes. It allows generating more than 250 decision rules of which 75 have been validated till now.

In the following example we trace the effect "appearance of a too low INR". When patients are under vitamin K antagonist (VKA) treatment, the international normalized ratio (INR) is traced in order to evaluate the treatment. In case of too high INR, there is a VKA overdose; the patient could present a hemorrhage. In case of too low INR, there is a VKA underdose; the patient is exposed to a risk of thrombosis. A tree is automatically generated.

The first split of the tree shows that the effect is most associated with the admission with a too high INR (risk of bleeding, Figure). When a patient enters the department with a too high INR there might be an over-correction of the treatment and a risk of thrombosis in 29% of the cases. Elderly patients admitted with a too high INR and a hypoalbuminemia are over-corrected in 87% cases. Albumin is the blood protein to which VKAs are linked. Only the unlinked fraction of VKAs is biologically active. Hypoalbuminemia was probably the cause of the too high INR but it also increases the effect of VKA correction, which was probably ignored by the physician.

That rule is interesting because it mixes together three kinds of conditions:

- a pharmacokinetics condition: hypoalbuminemia
- an epidemiological condition: the age

- an organizational condition: entry with too high INR

The patients who enter with a normal INR and receive in the same time VKA and a digestive prokinetic drug experience a too low INR in 67% cases (Figure a). Digestive prokinetic drugs decrease the bio-availability of VKA.

The patients aged less than 76 that are given VKA and beta lactam antibiotics experience a too low INR in 60% cases (Figure b). Several interpretations are possible: the antibiotic indicates an infection; infections may increase hepatic catabolism and decrease VKA bio-availability. Otherwise, antibiotics decrease vitamin K production in the digestive tract, that effect might be known and overbalanced by the physician.

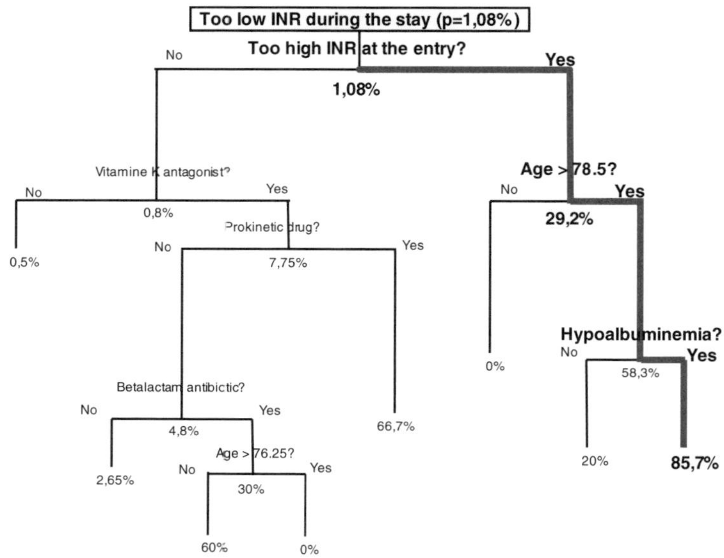

Figure 6. First rule gives p(too low INR during stay)=86% instead of 1%

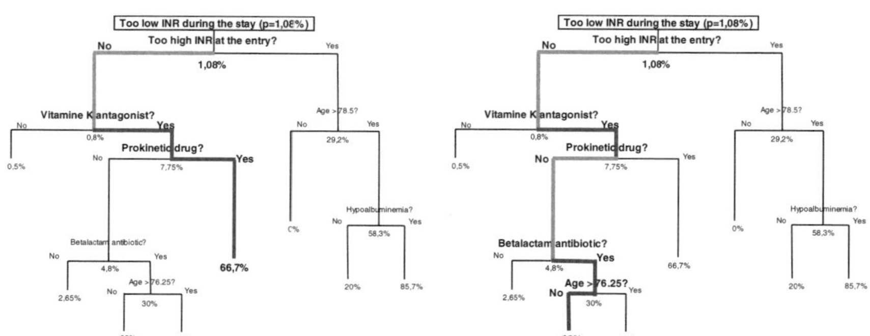

Figure 7. Second and third rules give p(too low INR during stay)= 67% and 80%

3. Discussion and Conclusion

Data mining often relies on a simple idea:

1. The observed effect is known: the group with effect (ADE=1) and the group without effect (ADE=0) have already been identified.
2. Several potential causes are available. In epidemiological projects, a restricted list of cause variables is chosen *a priori*. In data mining projects, a large set of potential causes is available; a statistical method is used to find the more significant ones.
3. The appropriate methods are used to explain the effect by the causes

That procedure is not possible in our project:

- mostly because *the effect is not identified*: no one flagged the cases as "normal" (ADE=0) nor "abnormal" (ADE=1), and our objective is to avoid a time-consuming staff operated review
- even most of the causes do not formally exist in the data

For that reason, data aggregation is a very important step. The accuracy of the results essentially relies on that step. However we are aware that despite its advantages, our procedure also suffers from some weaknesses. (1) Only the data that are recorded can be mined. Some clinical events might occur and might not be encoded in the EHR. (2) Diagnosis codes are important to describe acute and chronic diseases. Till now we are only able to take into account chronic diseases and acute diseases that cannot occur during the hospitalization. For instance if an ICD10 code describing a hemorrhage is present in the data, we cannot know if it is the admission ground or an event occurring during the hospitalization.

At the opposite of academic knowledge, the results of the PSIP project allow to sort the knowledge according to the probability of the events. For instance the "contraindication" and "use caution" sections of the French summaries of products characteristics of current VKAs are 3,300 words long. Moreover the knowledge that first appears in the text is already well known by the physicians so that the events that are first described rarely occur. The readers are flooded.

In addition, the rules from the PSIP project are able to take into account "what happened today". Conditions such as "the patient entered with a too high INR" are typically useful but absent from academic knowledge. Organizational circumstances are probably not enough considered.

First results of the PSIP project are encouraging [22] and announce a new approach in the ADE studies, actual approaches being essentially based on staff operated cases reviews [23] or databases queries [24-26]. The project is still be continued: the mapping policies are improved, the rule discovery is extended to other drugs and diseases, and other data-mining methods are being tried and compared with the decision trees: we are currently working on association rules [27, 28].

Acknowledgement

The research leading to these results has received funding from the European Community's Seventh Framework Program (FP7/2007-2013) [29, 30] under Grant Agreement n° 216130 - the PSIP project [3].

References

[1] Morimoto T, Gandhi TK, Seger AC, Hsieh TC, Bates DW. Adverse drug events and medication errors: detection and classification methods. Qual Saf Health Care. 2004 Aug;13(4):306-14.

[2] Murff HJ, Patel VL, Hripcsak G, Bates DW. Detecting adverse events for patient safety research: a review of current methodologies. J Biomed Inform. 2003 Feb-Apr;36(1-2):131-43.

[3] Patient Safety by Intelligent Procedures in medication. [cited 2009 february 24]; Available from: http://www.psip-project.eu.

[4] Adriaans P, Zantinge D, Syllogic (Firm). Data mining. Harlow, England ; Reading, Mass.: Addison-Wesley; 1996.

[5] Gurwitz JH, Field TS, Harrold LR, Rothschild J, Debellis K, Seger AC, et al. Incidence and preventability of adverse drug events among older persons in the ambulatory setting. JAMA. 2003 Mar 5;289(9):1107-16.

[6] Jalloh OB, Waitman LR. Improving Computerized Provider Order Entry (CPOE) usability by data mining users' queries from access logs. AMIA Annu Symp Proc. 2006:379-83.

[7] International Classification of Diseases. [cited 2009 february 24]; Available from: http://www.who.int/classifications/icd/en.

[8] Anatomical and Therapeutical Classification. [cited 2009 february 24]; Available from: http://www.whocc.no/atcddd.

[9] International Union of Pure and Applied Chemistry. [cited 2009 february 24]; Available from: http://www.iupac.org.

[10] Breiman L. Classification and regression trees. Belmont, Calif.: Wadsworth International Group; 1984.

[11] Fayyad U, Piatetsky-Shapiro G, Smyth P, editors. From data mining to knowledge discovery : an overview. 2nd Int Conf on Knowledge Discovery and Data Mining; 1996.

[12] Lavrac N. Selected techniques for data mining in medicine. Artif Intell Med. 1999 May;16(1):3-23.

[13] Quinlan JR. Introduction of Decision Trees. Machine Learning. 1986;1:81-106.

[14] Zhang HP, Crowley J, Sox H, Olshen RA. Tree structural statistical methods. Encyclopedia of Biostatistics. Chichester, England: Wiley; 2001. p. 4561-73.

[15] Ripley BD. Pattern recognition and neural networks. Cambridge ; New York: Cambridge University Press; 1996.

[16] Therneau TM, Atkinson B, Ripley B. rpart: Recursive Partitioning. 2007.

[17] R_Development_Core_Team. R: A Language and Environment for Statistical Computing. Vienna, Austria: R Foundation for Statistical Computing; 2008.

[18] Pharmacorama. [cited 2009 february 24]; Available from: http://www.pharmacorama.com.

[19] Banque de Données Automatisée sur les Médicaments. [cited 2009 february 24]; Available from: http://www.biam2.org/accueil.html.

[20] Theriaque. [cited 2009 february 24]; Available from: http://www.theriaque.org/InfoMedicaments.

[21] Pubmed. [cited 2009 february 24]; Available from: http://www.ncbi.nlm.nih.gov/pubmed.

[22] Beuscart R, Beuscart-Zéphir MC, the_PSIP_Consortium, editors. Workshop on Patient Safety through Intelligent Procedures in Medication. MIE Conference; 2008 25-28 May; Goteborg, Sweden.

[23] Bates DW, Evans RS, Murff H, Stetson PD, Pizziferri L, Hripcsak G. Detecting adverse events using information technology. J Am Med Inform Assoc. 2003 Mar-Apr;10(2):115-28.

[24] Honigman B, Lee J, Rothschild J, Light P, Pulling RM, Yu T, et al. Using computerized data to identify adverse drug events in outpatients. J Am Med Inform Assoc. 2001 May-Jun;8(3):254-66.

[25] Honigman B, Light P, Pulling RM, Bates DW. A computerized method for identifying incidents associated with adverse drug events in outpatients. Int J Med Inform. 2001 Apr;61(1):21-32.

[26] Seger AC, Jha AK, Bates DW. Adverse drug event detection in a community hospital utilising computerised medication and laboratory data. Drug Saf. 2007;30(9):817-24.

[27] Agrawal R, Imielinski T, Swami A, editors. Mining Association Rules between Sets of Items in Large Databases. Proceedings of the ACM SIGMOD International Conference on Management of Data; 1993 May. Washington D.C.

[28] Piatetsky-Shapiro G. Discovery, Analysis, and Presentation of Strong Rules. In: Frawley GP-SaWJ, editor. Knowledge Discovery in Databases. Cambridge, MA: AAAI/MIT Press; 1991.

[29] European Research Council. [cited 2009 february 24]; Available from: http://erc.europa.eu.

[30] Seventh Framework programme. [cited 2009 february 24]; Available from: http://cordis.europa.eu/fp7/home_en.html.

Detection and Prevention of Adverse Drug Events
R. Beuscart et al. (Eds.)
IOS Press, 2009

doi:10.3233/978-1-60750-043-8-85

The Expert Explorer: A Tool for Hospital Data Visualization and Adverse Drug Event Rules Validation

Adrian BĂCEANU [a, 1], Ionuţ ATASIEI [a], Emmanuel CHAZARD [b], Nicolas LEROY [b] and the PSIP Consortium [2]
[a] *Ideea Advertising, Bucharest, Romania*
[b] *Lille University Hospital, France*

Abstract. An important part of adverse drug events (ADEs) detection is the validation of the clinical cases and the assessment of the decision rules to detect ADEs. For that purpose, a software called "Expert Explorer" has been designed by Ideea Advertising. Anonymized datasets have been extracted from hospitals into a common repository. The tool has 3 main features. (1) It can display hospital stays in a visual and comprehensive way (diagnoses, drugs, lab results, etc.) using tables and pretty charts. (2) It allows designing and executing dashboards in order to generate knowledge about ADEs. (3) It finally allows uploading decision rules obtained from data mining. Experts can then review the rules, the hospital stays that match the rules, and finally give their advice thanks to specialized forms. Then the rules can be validated, invalidated, or improved (knowledge elicitation phase).

Keywords. Data Mining, Association rules, Database, Knowledge Elicitation, Web application.

Introduction

Adverse Drug Events (ADEs) endanger patients' safety and instigate considerable extra hospital costs [1]. Therefore, a significant reduction of preventable ADEs is a challenging issue in Public Health. Electronic health records (EHRs) seem to be the best information source in the field of ADEs detection and prevention [2, 3].

The PSIP project (Patient Safety through Intelligent Procedures in medication) [4] follows two main objectives:

- To produce epidemiological knowledge on Adverse Drug Events
- To design a clinical decision support system (CDSS) implementing some ADE detection rules, those rules being deduced from data mining [5] of the structured hospital data bases, and semantic mining of free text collections (e.g. discharge letters) [6].

As a part of the project, an EHR visualization tool has been required. A software called "Expert Explorer" has been designed to meet the following requirements:

[1] Corresponding author: Adrian Băceanu, Ideea Advertising, P-ta Mihail Kogalniceanu nr 1 bl 1 sc C ap 5, 050064, Bucuresti, Romania; Email: adrian.baceanu@ideea.biz

[2] CHRU Lille F, CHU Rouen F, CH Denain F, Region H Hospitals of Copenhagen DK, Oracle® F, IBM-Acure® DK, Medasys® F, Vidal® F, Ideea-Advertising® Ro, Kite® I, Aalborg University DK, Aristotle University of Thessaloniki GR, Umit Innsbruck A

- **Hospital stay display:** the tool must be able to display a given hospital stay thanks to visual and comprehensive pages. This visualization tool must display medical and administrative information including diagnoses and procedures, drug prescriptions, lab results, and reports (e.g. discharge letters).
- **Dashboards:** the tool must allow for dashboards design, execution and display. These dashboards will be used to provide on the fly epidemiological information about ADEs in each medical department.
- **Rules review and validation:** the tool must allow implementing the decision rules provided by the data-mining team. Once a rule is implemented, the Experts must be able to review all the hospital stays that match the rule and to fill an evaluation form. The results will be used to validate or not the rule. The rules-review tool uses the hospital-stay-display feature.

Moreover, the tool must respect some common requirements:

- The tool must be usable for every member of the research project, some users being able to connect from another country to a hospital database.
- Anonymity and confidentiality of the datasets are mandatory.

1. Available Data

In a first phase of the PSIP project, the available databases were identified and a generic access mechanism to the different data sources was developed. This was done by proposing and validating a common data model to extract data from the hospital databases, organize them under the same format, send them through FTP protocol, and prepare them for the next data (or semantic) mining phase.

A common data scheme (Figure) was agreed between partners to conduct data extraction from the various existing data [7].

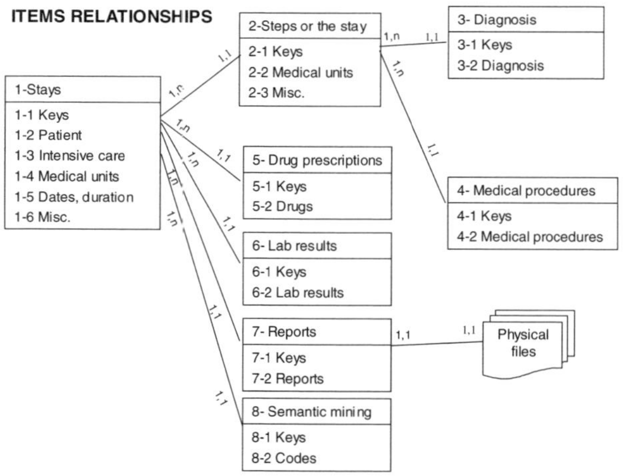

Figure 1. Simplified data scheme

The first extractions and exports of data were realized. The four data sources available to PSIP provided data as following:

- Some complete datasets, including patient description diagnoses and procedures (EHR), lab results (laboratory database) and drug prescriptions (Computer physician order entry CPOE):
  - o The Capital Region of Denmark Hospitals (RegionH hospitals, Dk) provided 2,600 hospital stays of year 2007 from cardiology and gerontology departments.
  - o The Denain hospital provided 10,000 hospital stays of year 2007 from surgery and medicine units
- Some incomplete datasets coming from hospitals without any CPOE. In those hospitals, information about drugs has been extracted from discharge letters thanks to semantic-mining:
  - o The Rouen university hospital provided 800 complete records. Its EHRs contain 1.4 million hospital stays and 5.3 million reports.
  - o The Lille university hospital has provided 10,000 records. Its EHR contains 2 millions patients and 20 millions reports and letters.

All the medical data have been anonymized and collected in a common repository. An important data management phase has been performed to ensure the quality of the data. This repository is completely anonymous and no personal information can be retrieved. Scripts have been written to make easier the data extraction. They can be re-utilised as frequently as necessary during the next steps of the project.

2. The Expert Explorer

2.1. General Presentation

One of the available solutions to have a data visualization tool, was the Oracle Business Intelligence Suite (OBI) [8], but the requirements that were formulated for this tool determined us to develop a custom solution: we needed a tool to work specially with the PSIP data model, we needed a more operational view, a tool that could generate laboratory results charts, drug charts, a tool that could allow different users to access the data and fill questionnaires to evaluate the hospital stays, a tool easy to use and focused on the goal it was designed for.

The Expert Explorer is a web-based data visualization tool. It allows representing several data from a given hospital stay: medical and administrative information, diagnoses, medical procedures, lab results and drug prescriptions. The application also offers a general overview of the medical department. The medical personnel can identify particular cases in the medical unit they have in charge. This is done by some primary statistics such as death rate, distribution by patient sex or the percent of hospital stays that implied an ICU. The user can generate reports based on the available details of the hospital stay. He can target specific values of the variables, and see the distribution of the stays in percent or mean values. The application is also a tool used as a support for evaluating the rules defined in the data and semantic mining process.

Using Expert Explorer one can apply primary statistics on the existing data sets: generate reports, update data sets used in the application, define rules and load rules from files, see the details of the hospital stays corresponding to the rules.

The Expert Explorer allows for several tasks:

- report generation: reports design using basic statistics, report publication

- visualization of the hospital stays from various datasets
- rules import: the rules can be then executed as SQL queries
- validation of the hospital stays obtained from data-mining: the expert can view the rules and the related stays, and validate them (or not) using a pre defined questionnaire.

2.2. Implementation and Availability

Expert Explorer is hosted on a web server and is available to anyone that knows the login credentials.

Data is stored using a MySQL [9] database and it uses the structure of the 8 tables structure defined during the first phase of the project.

The users that access the application can fit three different profiles: (1) general users, or guests that don't need a password, (2) medical experts that should login with a username and password and (3) administrators.

2.3. Data Sets Management

Before any activity, the user should choose the data set that he wants to work on. Also, on the same page (Figure) with data set selection, depending on his rights the users can update the data set, by uploading to the server the corresponding files.

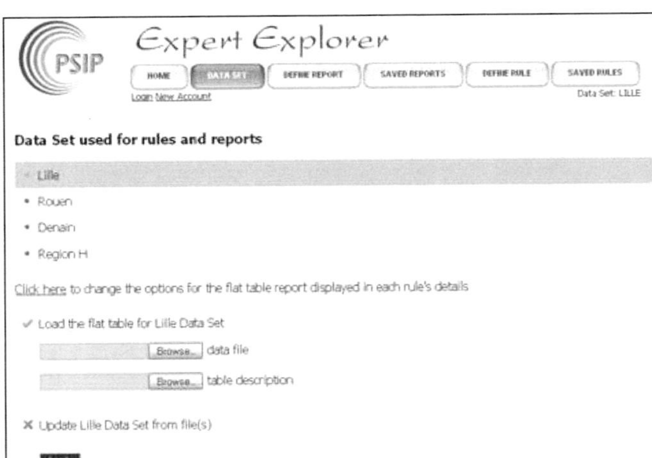

Figure 2. The page containing Data Set options

2.4. Reports Management

Reports definition and visualization was one of the firsts task designed in the Expert Explorer. The reports embed some basic statistical operations (count, mean…). The aim is to provide the physicians a comprehensive look over the patients they take care of.

The report has a table structure. The fields to use as lines labels are in fact selection fields for only the hospital stays that fit the selected value (WHERE SQL clauses) and aggregation fields (GROUP BY SQL clauses). The fields to use as columns are the fields to be aggregated (sums, counts, means…). As an example, the Death=1 can be used as a line label to restrict the dataset to hospital stays with death. At the opposite, the Mean (Death) can be used as a column label in order to compute the proportion of death in each subgroup. For this example, we have chosen sex and age as column labels and so there will a report for the hospital stays where the patient died, with details on the distribution in percent by sex and age.

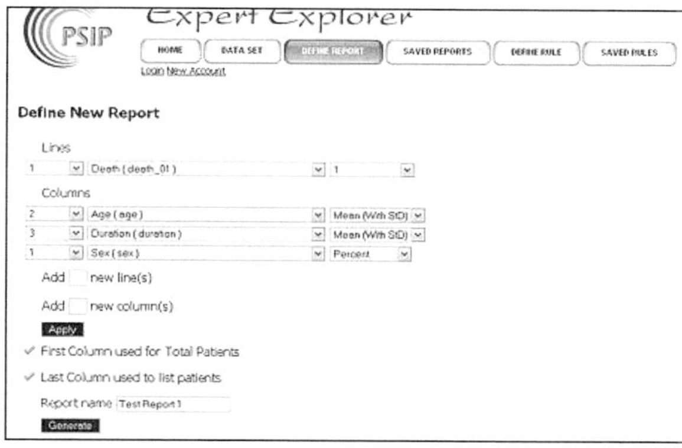

Figure 3. Defining a new report

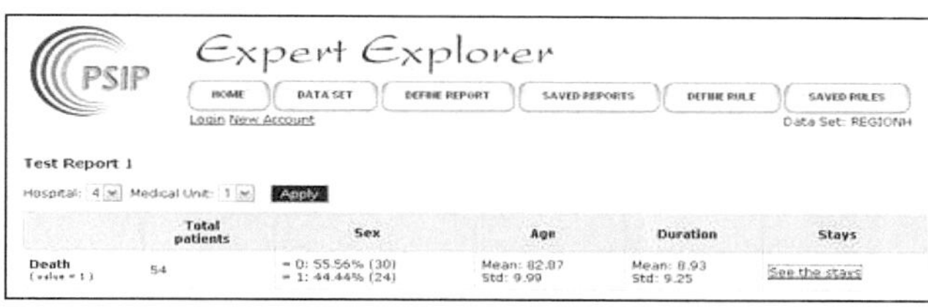

Figure 4. Visualisation of an already defined report

The report is displayed (Figure) using the table constructed when it was defined, with options to sort the table with a click on the columns names. When the option "Last column used to list patients" is checked, a link to a page that is listing all the hospital stays that match the report's criteria appears in the last column.

2.5. ADE Detection Rules Management

This section is used to define ADE detection rules. The rules can be defined manually or any file meeting the data-mining-team XML format can be directly uploaded.

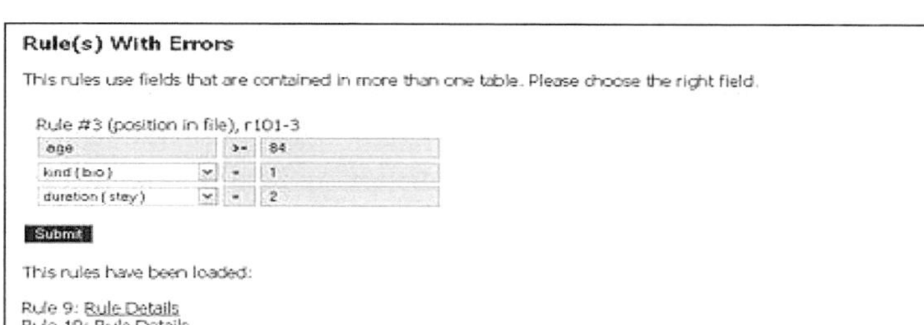

Figure 5. Correcting fields that weren't automatically matched in database

The rules use a structured formalism looking like "IF A1 AND A2 AND ... THEN B". This is not a natural language form. Only the fields existing in the tables can be used in a rule. The logical operator "and" and the usual comparison operators can be used. To define a rule, we select the field, the operator and the value on which the operator will be used. After defining a rule, it is kept in the database.

Using the "Import rule(s) from file" option the user can load rules from an external file. If there are two fields in different tables with the same name, the user will be asked to choose the correct field. (e.g. In Figure the fields "kind" and "stay" are present in two different tables).

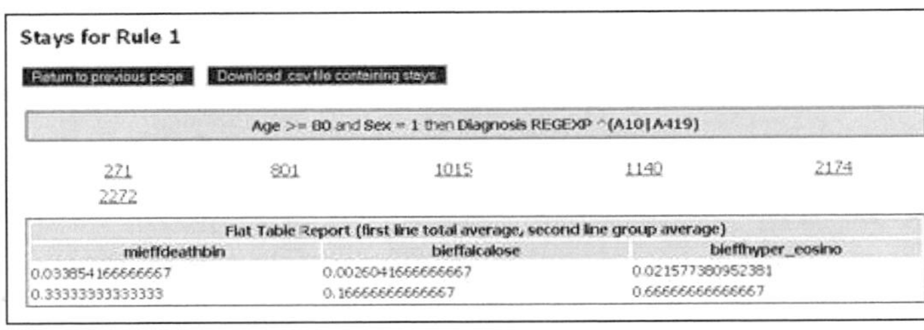

Figure 6. Details of a rule and the related hospital stays

The rule details page will display all the hospital stays that match this rule (Figure). Below the list of the stays returned by the rule, is a report based on an aggregated flat table. The columns used are defined on the Data Set page. The first line is an average of all the values from the flat table, for each column, the second line compute the averages only for the values associated to the group of hospital stays returned by the rule. A click on a hospital-stay identifier will bring up the page with all the details for that stay.

2.6. Visualization of a hospital stay

A hospital stay can be visualized in several contexts:

- As a standalone feature, the users are allowed to review every stays.
- Every implemented rule is associated to a report which displays links to the hospital stays that match the rule (Figure).

On the stay details page are displayed all the information available for that stay. The user only has to click on the desired tab. The following tabs are available:

- The first tab displays a description of the hospital stay (demographics, principal diagnosis, length of stay, etc.) (Figure)
- The second tab displays the different steps of the hospital stay, each step corresponding to a medical unit visited during the hospital stay.
- The third tab displays the medical procedures performed during the step of the hospital stay.
- The fourth tab shows the ICD10 diagnoses
- Another tab displays the drug administrations on a tabular form, and another tab presents that information in a comprehensive way thanks to a specific chart (Figure).
- The lab results can be displayed in a tabular form or thanks to a specific chart (Figure)

- Finally, it is possible to read all the anonymized reports free text documents (eg : discharge letter).

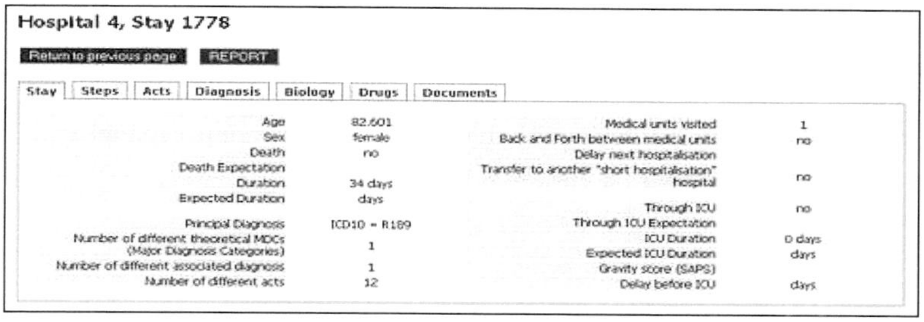

Figure 7. Hospital stay details page

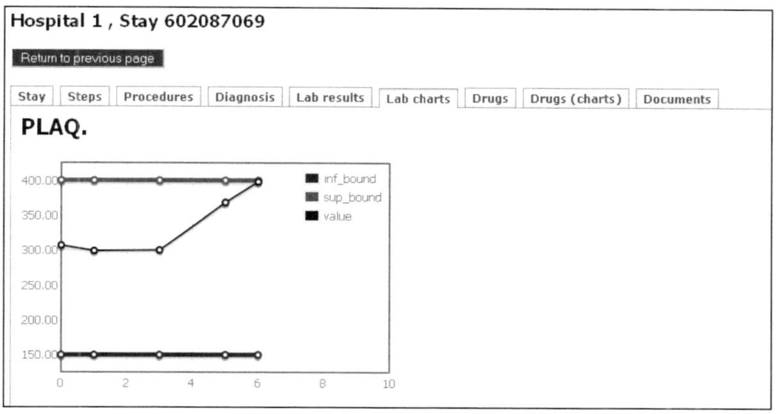

Figure 8. Lab-result-chart tab

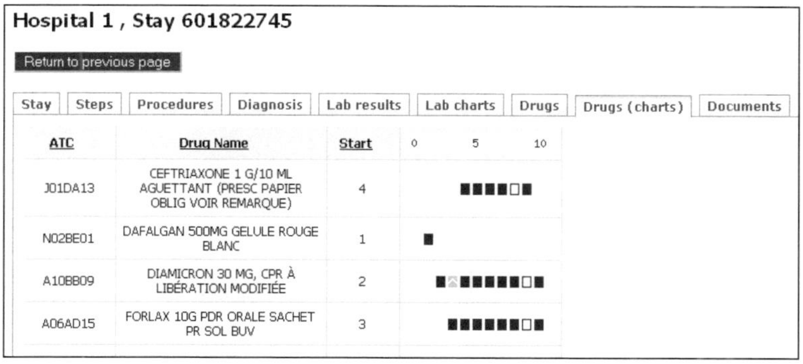

Figure 9. Drug-chart tab

2.7. User Account

The program is structured on three user levels of access, depending on the rule:

- Users (everybody) – can see/visualize data without having the power to modify them; can design and visualize dashboards
- Experts – can see/visualize and interpret the data; as a result to this he may register his advice and validate or invalidate the rules

- Administrator – has total access, the main role being that of implementing new rules and assign them for review; the administrator would also be in charge of updating the database's content

2.8. Experts' Rule Validation Task

When an expert logs in, he is presented with a personal control panel (Figure) that displays him the hospital stays he has to review.

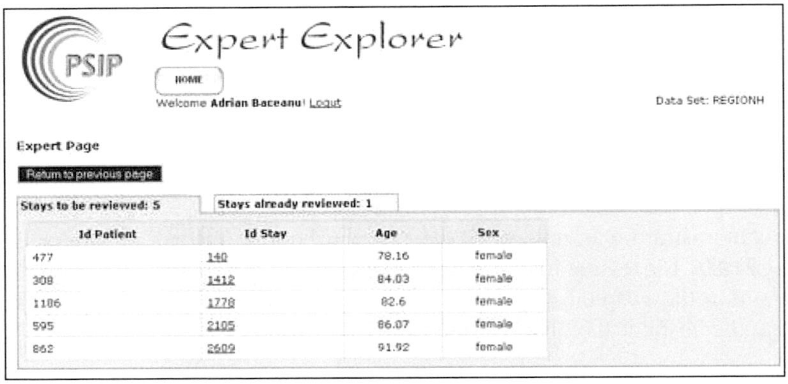

Figure 10. Expert's home page after login

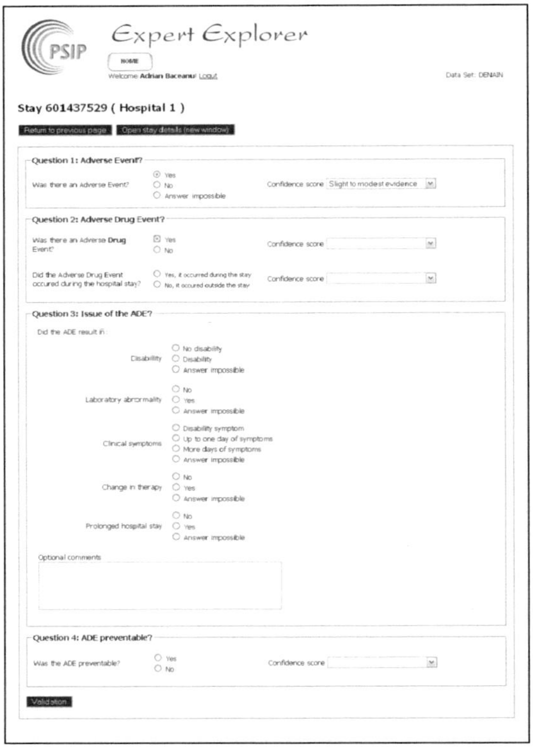

Figure 11. The pre defined questionnaire that the experts have to complete

The expert's home page contains two tabs: one where are listed the hospital stays that the expert need to review, and another with the hospital stays already reviewed. The expert can review the details of each particular stay and he can go to the report page where the pre defined questionnaire (Figure) can be completed, in order to determine if it was or wasn't an ADE.

The expert is asked, one at the time, several questions. Depending on the answer, the next question is displayed. He only has to select the answer, confidence score and sometimes he'll need to write personal comments. The expert can review a hospital stay, even if it is not associated with a rule. If the hospital stay has a rule associated, then two additional questions about the rule are displayed. If the expert already reviewed that hospital stay, then the questionnaire is automatically filled with his previous answers, and he has the option to modify his answers, or cancel and go to previous page.

Additional interactive functions allow supporting the reviewing process itself, allowing the experts to display the list of cases to be reviewed, to navigate through the data and to document the ADE Analysis form simultaneously.

The administrator can review all the expert accounts. The administrator is the one that assign rules for review to the experts. This can be done either by uploading a text file containing the hospital stay ids or by going through the previously defined rules and assign the hospital stay that the rules have returned.

3. Conclusion

Expert Explorer is developed exclusively based on the requirements from partners from the extraction phase, the data-mining phase, and finally the knowledge elicitation phase. It's currently subject to continuous updates.

Regarding the future evolution of Expert Explorer, we plan to improve it by implementing a module capable to automatically generate statistic rules. These automatically generated rules will be available to users only after they are approved by medical personnel. But this software main interest will be data visualization, data and semantic produced rules integration and data validation. Positive feedback from some of our partners and also from medical personnel that used the tool showed that it is a useful tool. We are convinced that, if it is used correctly, it may contribute in a significant way to the quality of medical services.

Some of the weak points of the tool include right now the use of a MySQL database and the server it is hosted on. When the volume of data will get bigger, a problem of updating the database can be issued. But to solve it, we aim towards the use of Oracle database. Oracle has many years of development and releases. Their tools (pl/sql, analytical functions, bulk loading, imports, exports, etc.) are far more advanced than any other database system out there [10].

A server hosting centralized data repository, managed by or just running Oracle solutions, could be of great use, because the tool could then only connect to that specific server and select the needed data.

The tool also lacks some evaluation: it is developed while integrating the point of view of ergonomic specialists, but regularly reviews of Expert Explorer take place.

Acknowledgment

The research leading to these results has received funding from the European Community's Seventh Framework Program (FP7/2007-2013) [11, 12] under grant agreement n°216130 - the PSIP project [4].

References

[1] Kohn LT, Corrigan J, Donaldson MS. To err is human : building a safer health system. Washington, D.C.: National Academy Press; 2000.
[2] Gurwitz JH, Field TS, Harrold LR, Rothschild J, Debellis K, Seger AC, et al. Incidence and preventability of adverse drug events among older persons in the ambulatory setting. JAMA. 2003 Mar 5;289(9):1107-16.
[3] Jalloh OB, Waitman LR. Improving Computerized Provider Order Entry (CPOE) usability by data mining users' queries from access logs. AMIA Annu Symp Proc. 2006:379-83.
[4] Patient Safety by Intelligent Procedures in medication. [cited 2009 february 24]; Available from: http://www.psip-project.eu.
[5] Adriaans P, Zantinge D, Syllogic (Firm). Data mining. Harlow, England ; Reading, Mass.: Addison-Wesley; 1996.
[6] Beuscart R, Beuscart-Zephir M-C, Brender J, Chazard E, Darmoni S, Jensen S, et al. PSIP Periodic report2009 February 26.
[7] Bernard O, Koncar M, Sarfati J-C, Chazard E, Niès J. Structures and Data Models of the Data repositories available in the PSIP project2008 May 21.
[8] Oracle Business Intelligence. [cited 2009 April 21]; Available from: http://www.oracle.com/solutions/business_intelligence/index.html.
[9] MySQL. [cited 2009 April 22]; Available from: http://www.mysql.com/.
[10] Oracle database. [cited 2009 April 22]; Available from: http://www.oracle.com/database/index.html.
[11] European Research Council. [cited 2009 february 24]; Available from: http://erc.europa.eu.
[12] Seventh Framework programme. [cited 2009 february 24]; Available from: http://cordis.europa.eu/fp7/home_en.html.

Detection and Prevention of Adverse Drug Events
R. Beuscart et al. (Eds.)
IOS Press, 2009

doi:10.3233/978-1-60750-043-8-95

Application of the Apriori Algorithm for Adverse Drug Reaction Detection

M. H. KUO [a, 1], A. W. KUSHNIRUK [a], E. M. BORYCK I [a] and D. GREIG [a]
[a] *School of Health Information Science, University of Victoria, BC, Canada*

Abstract. The objective of this research is to assess the suitability of the Apriori association analysis algorithm for the detection of adverse drug reactions (ADR) in health care data. The Apriori algorithm is used to perform association analysis on the characteristics of patients, the drugs they are taking, their primary diagnosis, co-morbid conditions, and the ADRs or adverse events (AE) they experience. This analysis produces association rules that indicate what combinations of medications and patient characteristics lead to ADRs. A simple data set is used to demonstrate the feasibility and effectiveness of the algorithm.

Keywords. Data Mining, Adverse Drug Reactions, Pharmacovigilance

Introduction

In recent years data mining has received considerable attention as a tool that can be applied to pharmacovigilance. There are many perspectives on the use of data mining as a tool for the detection of ADRs using clinical data [1-7]. Various data mining algorithms such as the Proportional Reporting Ratio (PRR) [8], Multi-item Gamma Poisson Shrinker (MGPS) [9], Bayesian Confidence Propagation Neural Network (BCPNN) [10], Proportional Reporting Odds Ratios (PROR), Bayesian Binary Logistic Regression (BBR), Genetic Algorithm [11], have been used to analyze data from Pharmacovigilance reporting systems and other sources of health data (e.g. electronic health records) in order to improve drug safety surveillance. Among these, three of the most commonly used algorithms are PRR, MGPS, and BCPNN. PRR has already been incorporated into the routine surveillance activities of the Medications and Healthcare Products Regulatory Agency (MHRA) in the UK. MGPS has been used by US FDA to look for signals of serious adverse events. The WHO Uppsala Monitoring Center (WHO-UMC) has incorporated BCPNN into its routine pharmacovigilance activities.

Compared to traditional surveillance methods these algorithms are very effective in detecting one to one relationships between a particular drug and an ADR. However they still have a number of limitations associated with their use. They have a very limited ability to identify drug-drug interaction or combinations of drugs that cause ADRs. They are also limited in their ability to identify other factors beyond the drug involved that may contribute to an ADR, such as patient diagnosis, comorbid conditions, and patient characteristics such as age. These algorithms themselves are meant to be used on very large data sets (The US FDA's Adverse Event Reporting System contains more than 2.5 million ADR reports) and do not produce usable results for smaller data sets such as those that are present in regional health authorities [2].

[1] Corresponding Author: akuo@uvic.ca

The objective of our research is to study the use of the *Apriori* algorithm to address the above mentioned problems and improve ADR detection and therefore improve patient safety. Research literature that describes or discusses pharmacovigilance specific potentials and applications of *Apriori* algorithms is currently very scarce (none published in Medline/PubMed as of January 2009). We believe that this algorithm is a powerful tool that can be used to improve post marketing surveillance and prospective pharmacovigilance programs.

1. Research method

Association analysis has been used extensively in business to analyze customer transactions and to find associations between the products consumers purchase [12]. However, its application to heath data is relatively unexplored. We are working in partnership with the BC Cancer Agency, Canada, using data extracted from their electronic health record system. The data is arranged into 'transactions' which contain a set of data items focused around a specific event, object, or time period. For our research a transaction is a collection of information about a patient and the ADRs they experience over a short period of time. For example:

{Age: 40-49, male, Bevacizumab, Lenolidamide, Hypertension, Diarrhea, GI Bleed, Sinusitis}

From these transactions association rules are generated, which is an implication of the form $\mathrm{X} \rightarrow \mathrm{Y}$, where X and Y are disjoint subsets of all the possible data items. For example: $\{\mathrm{Bevacizumab, Age\,60\text{-}69}\} \rightarrow \{\mathrm{Hypertension, Diarrhea}\}$

The strength of the association rule can be measured by its *support* and *confidence* as follows:

Let $I = \{i_1, i_1, \cdots, i_m\}$ be a set of items and $X, Y \subset I$, then the support of an association pattern is defined as equation (1).

$$support(X \rightarrow Y) = P(X \cap Y) \qquad (1)$$

, and the confidence of the association pattern is defined as equation (2).

$$confidence(X \rightarrow Y) = \frac{support(X \cap Y)}{support(X)} \qquad (2)$$

Support determines how often the data items in a rule are present together in a transaction in a given data set and is simply the count of transactions that contain X and Y. Support is used to determine if a rule is of interest as high support indicates that the rule occurs often in the data. Confidence is used to determine the reliability of the inference made by the rule and is an estimate of the conditional probability of Y given X. It says "If X is present in a transaction, how likely is it that Y is also present".

These rules suggest a strong co-occurrence relationship between the given data item subsets. It should be noted however that these rules do not automatically imply causality in a relationship [12]. The generated rules must be studied further to determine if causality exists or if other factors not captured in the data are influencing the association. The generated rules with high support and confidence provide an important starting point for pharmacovigilance efforts and help direct investigation and research to associations that are likely to prove useful or important. Using brute force to generate and test all possible rules in a set of data is not feasible as the total number of possible rules for a data set that contains *d* data items is: $R = 3^d - 2^{d+1} + 1$.

A data set containing only 13 data items would require calculating the support and confidence for 1,577,940 rules. The *Apriori* algorithm was proposed by Agrawal and Strikant in 1994 [13] and pioneered the use of support based pruning to control the exponential growth of potential rules [12, 14]. The algorithm employs an iterative approach known as level-wise search, where *k*-itemsets are used to explore *(k+1)*-itemsets.

2. A Case Study

For this case study we use a simple data set (Figure 1) and set a minimum support count of 3 and minimum confidence of 75%.

Patient ID	**List of ADRs**	
	Drugs	**Side Effects/Adverse Events**
P101	*Bevacizumab, Lenolidamide*	*Hypertension, Diarrhoea , GI Bleeding, Confusion, Sinusitis*
P102	*Bevacizumab*	*Hypertension, Diarrhoea, Dysplasia*
P103	*Lenolidamide*	*Confusion, Sinusitis, Fatigue*
P104	*Mitoxantrone*	*Amenorrhoea, Diarrhoea*
P105	*Flutamide*	*Anaemia, Impotence*
P106	*Bevacizumab, Lenolidamide*	*Hypertension, GI Bleeding, Confusion, Sinusitis, Hyperglycemia*
P107	*Bevacizumab, Mitoxantrone*	*Hypertension, Diarrhoea , Dyspnea*
P108	*Lenolidamide, Flutamide*	*Confusion, Sinusitis, Anaemia*
P109	*Ifosfamide, Mitoxantrone*	*Impotence, Hyperglycemia*
P110	*Bevacizumab, Lenolidamide*	*Diarrhoea , GI Bleeding, Confusion, Sinusitis*
P111	*Bevacizumab*	*Hypertension, Diarrhoea*
P112	*Lenolidamide, Ifosfamide*	*Confusion, Fatigue, Neutropenia*
P113	*Bevacizumab, Mitoxantrone*	*Hypertension, Diarrhoea, Sinusitis*

Figure 1. A simple adverse drug reactions Database (ADRDB)

Step 1: Find the support count of all the individual data items (1-itemsets) and eliminate those with a count < 3. For the purpose of the case study we only investigate rules (X → Y) where X is a drug and Y is an ADR. The support count for drugs and adverse events are as follows.

Candidate 1-Itemsets (MinSup = 3)	
Drugs	**Support Count**
Bevacizumab	7
Lenolidamide	6
Mitoxantrone	4

Candidate 1-Itemsets (MinSup = 3)	
Adverse Events	**Support Count**
Hypertension	6
Diarrhoea	7
GI Bleeding	3
Confusion	6
Sinusitis	5

Step 2: Find the support count for all the two data item rules (2-itemsets) using only the data times left over from step 1 and eliminate those with a count < 3.

Candidate 2-Itemsets (MinSup = 3)	
Adverse Events	**Support Count**
{Bevacizumab, Hypertension}	6
{Bevacizumab, Diarrhoea}	6
{Bevacizumab, GI Bleeding}	3
{Bevacizumab, Confusion}	3
{Bevacizumab, Sinusitis}	4
{Lenolidamide, Diarrhoea}	3
{Lenolidamide, GI Bleeding}	3
{Lenolidamide, Confusion}	6
{Lenolidamide, Sinusitis }	5
{Mitoxantrone, Diarrhoea}	3

Step 3: Find the support count for all the three data item rules (3-itemsets) using only the 2-itemsets left over from step 2 and eliminate those with a count< 3.

Candidate 3-Itemsets (MinSup = 3)	
Adverse Events	**Support Count**
{Bevacizumab, Hypertension, Diarrhoea}	5
{Bevacizumab, Hypertension, Sinusitis}	3
{Bevacizumab, Confusion, Sinusitis}	3
{ Lenolidamide, Confusion, Sinusitis}	5
{ Bevacizumab, Lenolidamide, GI Bleed}	5
{ Bevacizumab, Lenolidamide, Confusion}	3
{ Bevacizumab, Lenolidamide, Sinusitis}	3

Step 4: Find the support count for all the four data item rules (4-itemsets) using only the 3-itemsets left over from step 3 and eliminate those with a count < 3

.

Candidate 4-Itemsets (MinSup = 3)	
Adverse Events	**Support Count**
{Bevacizumab, Lenolidamide, Confusion, Sinusitis}	3

Step 5: Calculate the confidence of all the possible rules for the remaining itemsets and eliminate those with confidence < 75%.

Candidate 2-Itemsets (MinSup = 3)	
Adverse Events	**Confidence**
{Bevacizumab} → {Hypertension}	6/7 = 86%
{Bevacizuma} → {Diarrhoea}	6/7 = 86%
{Lenolidamide} → {Confusion}	6/6 = 100%
{Lenolidamide} → {Sinusitis }	5/6 = 83%
{Mitoxantrone} → {Diarrhoea}	3/4 = 75%

Candidate3-Itemsets (MinSup = 3)	
Adverse Events	**Confidence**
{ Lenolidamide} → {Confusion, Sinusitis}	5/6 = 83%
{ Bevacizumab, Lenolidamide} → {GI Bleed}	3/3 = 100%
{ Bevacizumab, Lenolidamide} → {Confusion}	3/3 = 100%
{ Bevacizumab, Lenolidamide} → {Sinusitis}	3/3 = 100%

Candidate 4-Itemsets (MinSup = 3)	
Adverse Events	**Confidence**
{Bevacizumab, Lenolidamide} → {Confusion, Sinusitis}	3/3=100%

Step 6: Analyze the results. Applying the *Apriori* algorithm to this simple data set has yielded some interesting relationships in the data. For example, neither of the rules {Bevacizumab → GI Bleeding} or {Lenalidamide → GI Bleeding} appear in the high confidence 2-itemset rules, however the rule {Bevacizumab, Lenalidamide → GI Bleeding} has a confidence of 100%. This would seem to indicate that Bevacizumab and Lenalidamide in combination may lead to GI Bleeding.

It is also of value to analyze the efficiency of the algorithm. With the constraint that we only investigate rules (X → Y) where X is a drug and Y is an ADR there are a total of 253,921 possible rules.

$$\binom{5}{1}\times\left\{\binom{13}{1}+\binom{13}{2}+\cdots+\binom{13}{13}\right\}$$
$$+\binom{5}{2}\times\left\{\binom{13}{1}+\binom{13}{2}+\cdots+\binom{13}{13}\right\}+\ldots$$
$$+\binom{5}{5}\times\left\{\binom{13}{1}+\binom{13}{2}+\cdots+\binom{13}{13}\right\}=253{,}921$$

Using the *Apriori* algorithm resulted in calculating support and confidence for only 55 rules, 0.02% of the total possible.

3. Conclusion

Currently most pharmacovigilance and drug safety monitoring efforts occur in a drug's pre-marketing phase during clinical trials and are administered by the drug manufacturer. Existing post-marketing surveillance programs generally involve voluntary spontaneous reporting (passive monitoring) of ADRs by physicians to a centralized province/state or nationwide repository. This does not provide a complete picture of the drug's safety profile in the general population as many ADRs, especially less severe ones, may go unreported. There is also often no way to link the ADR to the patient's medical history data in order to determine factors beyond the drug involved that may have contributed to the adverse event. There is a lack of post-marketing safety surveillance programs, data, and tools that focus on the prospective collection of ADR information by the institutions that are caring for the patients and administering the drugs. We used the *Apriori* algorithm to perform association analysis on the characteristics and attributes of the patient, the drugs they are taking, their primary diagnosis and comorbid conditions, and the ADRs they experience. The algorithm generates association rules that have high levels of confidence and support. It is able to detect drug-drug interactions and identify the attributes of patients who are at risk for experiencing ADRs while taking medications.

References

[1] DuMouchel, W., Fram, D., Yang, X., Mahmoud, R. A., Grogg, A. L., Engelhart, E. L. & Ramaswamy, K. (2008). Antipsychotics, Glycemic Disorders, and Life-Threatening Diabetic Events: A Bayesian Data-Mining Analysis of the FDA Adverse Event Reporting System (1968-2004), Annals of Clinical Psychiatry, 20(1), 21–31.

[2] Matsushita Matsushita, Y., Kuroda, Y., Niwa, S., Sonehara, S., Hamada, C. & Yoshimura, I. (2007). Criteria Revision and Performance Comparison of Three Methods of Signal Detection Applied to the Spontaneous Reporting Database of a Pharmaceutical Manufacturer. Drug Safety; 30(8), 715-726.

[3] Hauben, M., Horn, S. & Reich, L. (2007). Potential Use of Data-Mining Algorithms for the Detection of 'Surprise' Adverse Drug Reactions. Drug Safety; 30(2), 143-155.

[4] Almenoff, J. S., LaCroix, K. K., Yuen, N. A., Fram, D. & DuMouchel, W. (2006). Comparative Performance of Two Quantitative Safety Signalling Methods - Implications for Use in a Pharmacovigilance Department. Drug Safety; 29(10), 875-87.

[5] Hauben, M., Patadia, V., Gerrits, C., Walsh, L. and Reich, L. (2005). Data Mining in Pharmacovigilance - The Need for a Balanced Perspective. Drug Safety; 28(10), 835-842.

[6] Hauben, M. & Zhou, X. (2003). Quantitative Methods in Pharmacovigilance. Drug Safety; 26(3), 159-186.

[7] Szarfman, A., Machado, S. G. & O'Neill, R. T. (2002). Use of Screening Algorithms and Computer Systems to Efficiently Signal Higher-Than-Expected Combinations of Drugs and Events in the US FDA's Spontaneous Reports Database. Drug Safety; 25(6), 381-392.

[8] Evans, S. J. W., Waller, P. C. & Davis, S. (2001). Use of proportional reporting ratios (PRRs) for signal generation from spontaneous adverse drug reaction reports. Pharmacoepidemiology. Drug Safety; 10, 483-86.

[9] DuMouchel, W. & Pregibon D. (2001). Empirical Bayes screening for multi-item associations. In: Conference on knowledge discovery in data. Proceedings of the Seventh ACM SIGKDD Inter national Conference on Knowledge Discovery and Data Mining; San Francisco (CA). New York: ACM Press, 67-76.

[10] Bate, A., Lindquist, M., Edwards, I.R., et al. (1998). A Bayesian neural network method for adverse drug reaction signal generation. Eur J Clin Pharmacol; 54, 315-21.

[11] Koh,Y., Yap, C. W. & Li, S.C. (2008). A quantitative approach of using genetic algorithm in designing a probability scoring system of an adverse drug reaction assessment system. International Journal of Medical Informatics, 7(7), 421–430

[12] Tan, P. N., Steinbach, M. & Kumar, V. (2006). Introduction to Data Mining. Addison-Wesley.

[13] Agrawal, R. & Srikant, R. (1994). Fast Algorithms for Mining Association Rules, VLDB, Proceedings of the 20th VLDB Conference, Santiago, Chile, 487-99.

[14] Kotsiantis, S. & Kanellopoulos, D. (2006). Association Rules Mining: A Recent Overview, GESTS International Transactions on Computer Science and Engineering. 32 (1), 71-82

Detection and Prevention of Adverse Drug Events
R. Beuscart et al. (Eds.)
IOS Press, 2009

doi:10.3233/978-1-60750-043-8-102

Adverse Drug Events Prevention Rules: Multi-site Evaluation of Rules from Various Sources

Emmanuel CHAZARD [a,1], Grégoire FICHEUR [a], Béatrice MERLIN [a], Elisabeth SERROT [b], the PSIP Consortium and Régis BEUSCART [a]
[a] *Lille university hospital, EA2694, France*
[b] *Vidal SA, France*

Abstract. Adverse drug events are a public health issue (98,000 deaths in the USA every year). Some computerized physician order entry (CPOEs) coupled with clinical decision support systems (CDSS) allow to prevent ADEs thanks to decision rules. Those rules can come from many sources: academic knowledge, record reviews, and data mining. Whatever their origin, the rules may induce too numerous alerts of poor accuracy when identically applied in different places. In this work we formalized rules from various sources in XML and enforced their execution on several medical departments to evaluate their local confidence. The article details the process and shows examples of evaluated rules from various sources. Several needs are enlightened to improve confidences: segmentation, contextualization, and evaluation of the rules over time.

Keywords. Adverse drug events, data mining, decision rules, XML, CPOE, CDSS.

Introduction

Adverse drug events (ADEs) are a public health issue: every year they are considered responsible for 10,000 deaths in France and 98,000 deaths in the USA [1] in both ambulatory care and hospitalization. During hospitalizations some ADEs can be prevented when a computerized provider order entry (CPOE) is the frame of the medication use process and is coupled with a clinical decision support system (CDSS). In those CDSS it is possible to implement some alert rules, e.g. when some drugs are prescribed despite a drug-drug or a drug-diagnosis contraindication. Many different methods allow generating alert rules, each method having some qualities and drawbacks in regard to formalism, confidence, segmentation, and generation hardness:

- Academic knowledge (e.g. summaries of products characteristics, pharmacology teaching, ADE declarations, clinical trials)
- Staff operated reviews (e.g. records reviews, charts reviews, expert reviews)
- Automated data mining (e.g. decision trees, association rules)

Each method has advantages and drawbacks. Three drawbacks seem to be often underestimated:

- **the lack of segmentation** (subgroups variations of the confidence):

[1] Corresponding Author: Dr Emmanuel Chazard, CHRU Lille, 2 avenue Oscar Lambret, 59000 Lille, France; E-mail: emmanuel@chazard.org.

A rule such as "drug_A => effect" might be always true, but its confidence depends on several other variables. Some conditions such as "age>70" or "renal insufficiency" could improve the confidence of the rule and then the interest of alerting the physicians:

$$P(effect) < P(effect \mid drug\_A) < P(effect \mid drug\_A \cap age>70)$$

prevalence < *confidence of the rule* < *confidence of the rule with segmentation*

- **the lack of contextualization** (transversal changes):
  Whatever their origin, rules are applied as they are in every medical department assuming that the same causes necessary lead to the same effects with a constant probability. But in fact the alerts are too numerous and their accuracy seems to strongly depend on the place. Though, depending on the medical department the patients could differ (gender, age, associated diseases), the indication of the same drug could vary, as well as the physicians' knowledge about drugs and their risk aversion.
- **the lack of over time evaluation** (longitudinal changes):
  We hope that good rules implemented into a CDSS coupled with a CPOE will improve the physicians' knowledge about drugs and their practices. Therefore the confidences of the rules will decrease and there will be an over-alerting risk. Only an iterative evaluation of the confidences could answer that problem.

The aim of the present work is to formalize different rules from various sources in a uniform way in order to feed a rules repository, and to be able for each rule to compute its confidence on the fly in different medical departments.

1. Material

1.1. Datasets for Rules Evaluation

Electronic Health Records (EHRs) seems to be the best data source in the field of ADEs [2, 3]. A data model has been designed in the context of PSIP. It contains 8 tables and 92 fields (Figure) and is used in a central repository.

Data extractions were performed to feed the repository. An important point is that no data has to be specifically recorded for the project: only widely available data are used. As a consequence, data extraction generalization and follow-up is much easier. These data include:

- medical and administrative information
- diagnoses encoded using ICD10 [4]
- medical procedures encoded using national classifications
- drug prescriptions encoded using the ATC classification [5]
- laboratory results encoded using the C-NPU classification (IUPAC) [6]

Data extraction is still being continued. The present work is realized on 10,500 complete hospital stays of year 2007 from Denmark and France, mostly from cardiologic or geriatric units:

- Capital Region of Denmark hospitals (Dk): 2,700 hospital stays
- Denain hospital (Fr): 7,000 hospital stays
- Rouen university hospital (Fr): 800 hospital stays. This hospital doesn't have any CPOE: that's the reason why its data cannot be used to generate rules.

However, as discharge letters could be semantically-mined, ATC codes found in the text can be used to replace data from CPOE. It is sufficient to allow for rules evaluation on the Rouen hospital stays.

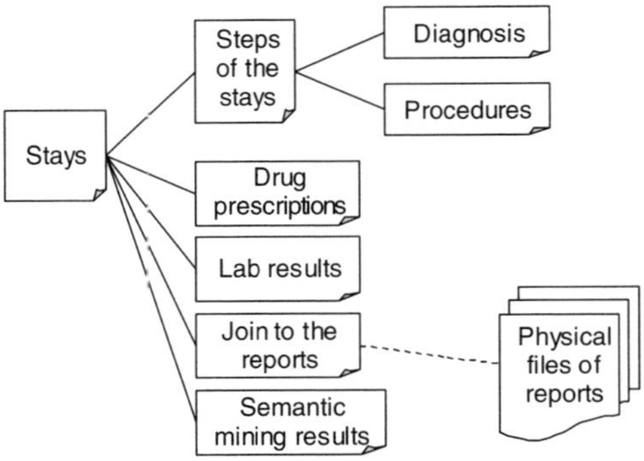

Figure 1. Simple view of the 8 tables of the data model.

1.2. Rules from Academic Knowledge

Vidal S.A. [7] is a French company that provides information about drugs and therapeutics. Vidal contents are used by almost all French physicians and also in different languages in others countries. Vidal's knowledge comes from official summaries of product characteristics, recent studies, official recommendations, literature, and experts' advice. Vidal contents and services include drug information, therapeutic guidelines and decision support modules. Being a partner of the PSIP project, the Vidal Company gives us access to formalized associations rules.

Their association rules provide four alert levels: absolute contra-indication, relative contra-indication, use caution, notice. The rules are built as follows: two causes brought together might induce one effect. The effect is expressed according to a proprietary thesaurus. The two causes can be of several kinds (but at least one of the conditions is a drug of a class of drug):

- drugs or classes of drugs
- classes of diagnoses
- creatinine clearance lower than a given threshold
- age, gender, pregnancy, allergies, breast feeding…

Advantages:

- That source provides all the "official" information.
- Even rare effects are mentioned.
- Even conditions that might never occur together appear (exhaustive list of absolute contra-indications).

Drawbacks:

- The number of rules is very high.
- Support and confidence (positive predictive values) of the rules are not provided (academic knowledge relies on clinical trials and spontaneous declarations that do not reflect the prevalence of ADEs [8, 9]).

- Many effects described by the rules are available in the EHRs (e.g. clinical events). Only some of the effects are usable in this work in view of which a mapping has to be realized.
- There are only and always two conditions per rule, no segmentation.
- There is no contextualization: the knowledge applies on a whole country

Integration of this knowledge in the repository:

- The rules are first restricted to absolute contra-indications.
- The rules are then limited to those where the effect can be traced in the database. Some approximations are done to trace some effects, e.g. "*drug_A => rhabdomyolysis*" is transformed into "*drug_A => hyperkaliemia & elevation of muscle enzymes & renal insufficiency*".

1.3. Rules from Expert Reviews

In a recent paper [10], Jah et al. published a list of 30 alerts from the VigiLanz commercial application. Those alerts are rules composed by a drug as the cause, and a lab alert. 10 of those alerts are validated as ADEs or potential ADEs.

Advantages:

- The rules are easy-to-implement, the effect is traceable.
- Rules have been validated by a staff operated record review.
- Confidence (positive predictive value) and support have been computed.

Drawbacks:

- The number of events is low.
- There is only and always one condition per rule, there is no segmentation.
- The rules are not contextualized.

Integration of this knowledge in the repository:

- The rules are implemented without any change in the rules repository.

1.4. Rules from Data Mining: Decision Trees

In the frame of the PSIP project [11] we analyzed 10,500 hospital stays. We computed decision trees [12-18] with the CART method thanks to the RPART package [19] of R [20]. The rules were computed separately on each medical department. The rules we obtained associate a variable number of conditions to a traceable effect and take chronology into account. The conditions can have various natures: a drug prescription, the presence of a group of ICD10 diagnoses, an acute or chronic lab abnormality, data about the patient (e.g. gender, age), data about the organizational conditions of the hospital stay (e.g. admission by emergency, with a too high INR, on Saturday, etc.)

Advantages:

- The rules can be automatically implemented: the same structured database is used for rules generation and for rules evaluation.
- Confidence (positive predictive value) and support have been computed.
- Each rule can consider a variable number of causes, from various natures (lab, drugs, diagnoses, patient, organizational causes).

- The population is segmented in order to optimize the confidence of the rules and to decreases over-alerting.
- The rules are contextualized: their confidence have been computed separately on each medical department

Drawbacks:

- Only events that are not too rare can be observed because a strong statistical link is required
- Only conditions that occur together can appear: absolute contra-indications should never appear although their implementation is mandatory
- Trees are known for their instability and the risk of omitting interesting rules

Integration of this knowledge in the repository:

- The rules are implemented without change in the rules repository. Only the rules that can be validated according to drug-related web information portals [21-23] and Pubmed [24] are used.

In the frame of the PSIP project we are now completing the data mining by using association rules [25, 26]. The aim is to discover some rules that could not appear using decision trees. Association rules produce a more exhaustive set of rules than decision trees. Those rules have to be filtered.

1.5. Rules Description and Storage in the Central Repository

The central rules repository is fed by several sources (Figure a):

- Automatic rules production from the Denain hospital (F) and the RegionH hospital (Dk), using data mining (decision trees and association rules) [11]
- Manual transformation of rules coming from foreign sources: academic knowledge (presently Vidal) and scientific articles (presently Jah et al.)

An XML [27] scheme has been conceived to represent the rules. XML is chosen because of the following characteristics:

- XML allows building semi-structured database: a complex data scheme with much cardinality can be defined much simpler than using relational databases. Any update of the scheme is easy too.
- XML can be easily produced by many programs. Our R scripts were modified to automatically generate XML in addition to standard output (Figure). During the test phase we were able to edit the data with only a simple text editor and to get preliminary results.
- XSL and XSL-FO transformation allows to quickly designing many kinds of outputs (e.g. text files, HTML, PDF, and XML). All the programming languages are able to load XML data to compute treatments that would be too complex for XSLT.
- A unique central repository can then be used to store all our knowledge about ADEs, including free text comments and bibliographic references

The XML data scheme contains two main parts: (1) the rules description (2) last available data about rules occurrences on every place (Figure).

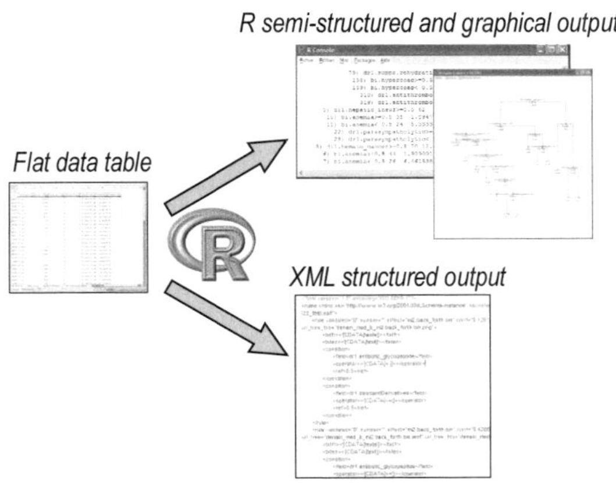

Figure 2. Automatic XML output of R scripts

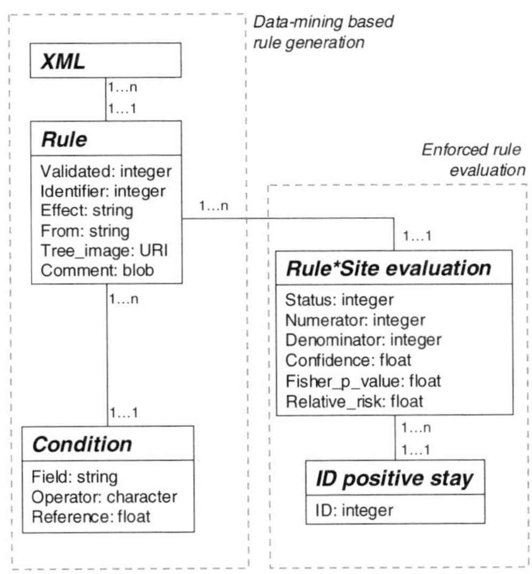

Figure 3. XML data scheme

1.6. Rules Evaluation

A rule is a set of causes leading to an effect, such as C_1 & C_2 & C_3=>E

In a few seconds, all the validated rules can be automatically evaluated on every medical department. The evaluation uses the 10,500 hospital stays from Denain (F), RegionH (Dk) and also Rouen (F) (Figure b). Rules enforced evaluation allows to add another knowledge into the database: rules occurrences. Then it is possible to answer several questions for each rule, separately in each medical department:

- Do some hospital stays match the conditions?
  number of stays = $\#(C_1 \cap C_2 \cap C_3)$
- Among those stays, do some hospital stays encounter the expected effect?
  number of stays = $\#(E \cap C_1 \cap C_2 \cap C_3)$
  support = $P(E \cap C_1 \cap C_2 \cap C_3)$
  confidence = $P(E \mid C_1 \cap C_2 \cap C_3)$

- What are the identifiers of the hospital stays that match the complete rule?
- Is it possible to quantify the strength of the association?
  relative risk = confidence / prevalence = $P(E \mid C_1 \cap C_2 \cap C_3) / P(E)$
  p value of the Fisher test comparing $P(E \mid C_1 \cap C_2 \cap C_3)$ *and* $P(E)$
- Are those patients similar to others? (Descriptive statistics only)
  on the subset $E \cap C_1 \cap C_2 \cap C_3$, *compute mean(gender), mean(age), etc.*
- What happens to those patients? (Descriptive statistics only)
  on the subset $E \cap C_1 \cap C_2 \cap C_3$, *compute mean(death), mean(duration , etc.*

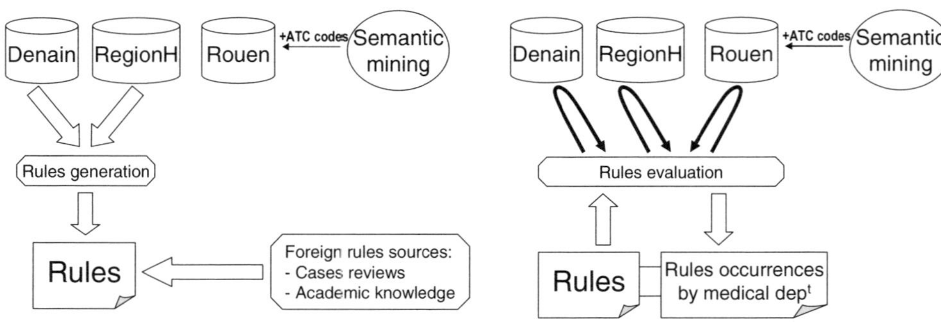

(a) rules production and incorporation *(b) rules enforced multi-site evaluation*

Figure 4. Rules centralization and enforced multi-site evaluation

2. Results

The mechanism properly works and the present task has to be carried on. Till now, rules centralization and evaluation use:

- 75 rules from data mining (rules were obtained from decision trees. Association rules exploitation has just began)
- about 100 rules from Vidal
- 30 rules from Jah et al.

Table presents nine rules that are interesting.

Rules Nr 1 & 2 are single condition rules that come from a staff operated review. It is interesting to notice that their confidences are low and vary from a medical department to another.

Rule Nr 3 comes from the same source and was also found as is by our decision trees. Decision trees are able to find that rule because the confidence is 33% in two departments. That confidence also varies according to the medical department.

Rules Nr 4, 5 & 6 help to understand what can happen when the confidence of academic rules is low. Rule Nr 4 & 5 come from the staff operated review, their confidence is low because the denominator is a too high number (their use would induce an over-alerting). Decision trees also allow finding rule Nr 6: that rules combines rules Nr 4 & 5 with other conditions so that the confidence is increased. Rule Nr 6 would have less false positives than rules Nr 4 or 5.

Rules Nr 7, 8 & 9 are generated by the data mining process. They are an interesting example of thinking about a prospective use of retrospective rules. Rules Nr 7 & 9 look the same except the third condition of each one: in rule Nr 7 there is a hypoalbuminemia and in rule Nr 9 there is no hypoalbuminemia. This third condition leads to different confidences in the departments, it is a segmentation condition. But in a prospective way it might be possible that this lab setting is still not available. However, we are able to answer the question "what is the probability of too low INR if we don't know the albumin blood rate". The answer is provided by rule Nr 8 where hypoalbuminemia=NA (not available), assuming that the lab result is missing at random.

Table 1. Example of rules and enforced evaluation results

Effect	id	Condition(s)	REGIONH	Denain Medicine A	Denain Medicine B	Denain Surgery	Rouen
Appearance of a renal insufficiency [Lab]	1	Histamine h2 antagonist	0/3=0%	2/15=13%	0/13=0%	0/4=0%	0/3=0%
	2	Non-steroidal anti-inflammatory agent	20/686=3%	15/393=4%	19/319=6%	3/217=1%	5/234=2%
	3	Antiviral agent	0/12=0%	1/3=33%	4/12=33%	0/1=0%	0/6=0%
	4	Heparin	17/445=4%	26/478=5%	34/473=7%	7/798=1%	1/50=2%
	5	Potassium lowering diuretic	46/841=5%	39/467=8%	25/297=8%	9/218=4%	5/260=2%
	6	Diuretic & Heparin & Age>75	3/32=9%	14/19=73%	9/19=47%	2/18=11%	0/0
Appearance of a too low inr [Lab]	7	Previous too high INR & Age>75 & Hypoalbuminemia	7/12=58%	2/2=100%	2/3=66%	2/7=29%	6/8=75%
	8	Previous too high INR & Age>75 & Unknown blood albumin level	8/20=40%	20/53=38%	15/26=58%	7/13=54%	8/11=73%
	9	Previous too high INR & Age>75 & NO hypoalbuminemia	1/8=12%	18/51=35%	13/23=56%	5/6=83%	2/3=66%

3. Discussion and Conclusion

Each of the various sources of ADE rules has its own characteristics. A comparison is provided in Table . Our conclusion is that an efficient rules repository should incorporate rules from various sources because of the advantages and drawbacks of each method.

This work enabled the uniform representation and storage of ADE detection rules into a common repository. Those rules can be then evaluated in a few seconds in several medical departments. This work has to be followed up in order to get more rules and more rules evaluations. However it already enlightens three major points that are often underestimated in ADE prevention rules:

- **the need for segmentation** in order to get more precise estimators of probabilities and to reduce over-alerting. Some of those segmentation conditions can also be "non medical" conditions such as organizational causes and human factors [11]

- **the need for contextualization**: whatever their origin, the rules do not have the same confidence everywhere
- **the need for an evaluation over time** of the rules over time: the existence of alert rules could quickly change the practices and then the confidences of the rules.

Table 2. General considerations about various sources of rules

Question	Academic knowledge	Staff operated record review	Data mining
Number of rules	Very high	Low	Medium
Need for validation	No, commonly accepted	Yes, already done in the process	Yes, must be performed, but sometimes difficult
Confidences of the rules	Not available	Computed by experts	Automatically computed
Number of the conditions	Few (1 or 2)	Depends on the review, often few	Variable, potentially high
Population segmentation, confidences optimization	No	No	Yes
Ability to propose rules when conditions never occur (e.g. absolute contra-indications)	Yes	No	No
Ability to describe very rare events	Yes	Sometimes possible	No
Ability to find all the interesting rules of a dataset	Yes	Yes but limited by the size of the review	Yes depending on the methods (association rules better than decision trees)
Time needed to find rules	Already available	Very time-consuming	Quite fast
Time needed to update confidences over space and times	Not possible	Very time-consuming	Very fast

Acknowledgement

The research leading to these results has received funding from the European Community's Seventh Framework Program (FP7/2007-2013) [28, 29] under Grant Agreement n° 216130 - the PSIP project [30].

References

[1] Kohn LT, Corrigan J, Donaldson MS. To err is human : building a safer health system. Washington, D.C.: National Academy Press; 2000.
[2] Gurwitz JH, Field TS, Harrold LR, Rothschild J, Debellis K, Seger AC, et al. Incidence and preventability of adverse drug events among older persons in the ambulatory setting. JAMA. 2003 Mar 5;289(9):1107-16.
[3] Jalloh OB, Waitman LR. Improving Computerized Provider Order Entry (CPOE) usability by data mining users' queries from access logs. AMIA Annu Symp Proc. 2006:379-83.
[4] International Classification of Diseases. [cited 2009 february 24]; Available from: http://www.who.int/classifications/icd/en.
[5] Anatomical and Therapeutical Classification. [cited 2009 february 24]; Available from: http://www.whocc.no/atcddd.
[6] International Union of Pure and Applied Chemistry. [cited 2009 february 24]; Available from: http://www.iupac.org.
[7] Vidal S.A. [cited 2009 April, 23]; Available from: http://www.vidal.fr/societe/vidal.
[8] Morimoto T, Gandhi TK, Seger AC, Hsieh TC, Bates DW. Adverse drug events and medication errors: detection and classification methods. Qual Saf Health Care. 2004 Aug;13(4):306-14.
[9] Murff HJ, Patel VL, Hripcsak G, Bates DW. Detecting adverse events for patient safety research: a review of current methodologies. J Biomed Inform. 2003 Feb-Apr;36(1-2):131-43.
[10] Jha AK, Laguette J, Seger A, Bates DW. Can surveillance systems identify and avert adverse drug events? A prospective evaluation of a commercial application. J Am Med Inform Assoc. 2008 Sep-Oct;15(5):647-53.
[11] Chazard E, Preda C, Merlin B, Ficheur G, Beuscart R. Data-mining-based detection of adverse drug events. Stud Health Technol Inform. 2009;[IN PRESS].
[12] Breiman L. Classification and regression trees. Belmont, Calif.: Wadsworth International Group; 1984.
[13] Fayyad U, Piatetsky-Shapiro G, Smyth P, editors. From data mining to knowledge discovery : an overview. 2nd Int Conf on Knowledge Discovery and Data Mining; 1996.
[14] Lavrac N. Selected techniques for data mining in medicine. Artif Intell Med. 1999 May;16(1):3-23.
[15] Piatetsky-Shapiro G, Frawley W. Knowledge discovery in databases. Menlo Park, Calif.: AAAI Press : MIT Press; 1991.
[16] Quinlan JR. Introduction of Decision Trees. Machine Learning. 1986;1:81-106.
[17] Ripley BD. Pattern recognition and neural networks. Cambridge ; New York: Cambridge University Press; 1996.
[18] Zhang HP, Crowley J, Sox H, Olshen RA. Tree structural statistical methods. Encyclopedia of Biostatistics. Chichester, England: Wiley; 2001. p. 4561-73.
[19] Therneau TM, Atkinson B, Ripley B. rpart: Recursive Partitioning. 2007.
[20] R_Development_Core_Team. R: A Language and Environment for Statistical Computing. Vienna, Austria: R Foundation for Statistical Computing; 2008.
[21] Pharmacorama. [cited 2009 february 24]; Available from: http://www.pharmacorama.com.
[22] Banque de Données Automatisée sur les Médicaments. [cited 2009 february 24]; Available from: http://www.biam2.org/accueil.html.
[23] Theriaque. [cited 2009 february 24]; Available from: http://www.theriaque.org/InfoMedicaments.
[24] Pubmed. [cited 2009 february 24]; Available from: http://www.ncbi.nlm.nih.gov/pubmed.
[25] Agrawal R, Imielinski T, Swami A, editors. Mining Association Rules between Sets of Items in Large Databases. Proceedings of the ACM SIGMOD International Conference on Management of Data; 1993 May. Washington D.C.
[26] Piatetsky-Shapiro G. Discovery, Analysis, and Presentation of Strong Rules. In: Frawley GP-SaWJ, editor. Knowledge Discovery in Databases. Cambridge, MA: AAAI/MIT Press; 1991.
[27] eXtensible Markup Language. [cited 2009 April, 23]; Available from: http://www.w3.org/XML/.
[28] European Research Council. [cited 2009 february 24]; Available from: http://erc.europa.eu.
[29] Seventh Framework programme. [cited 2009 february 24]; Available from: http://cordis.europa.eu/fp7/home_en.html.
[30] Patient Safety by Intelligent Procedures in medication. [cited 2009 february 24]; Available from: http://www.psip-project.eu.

Detection and Prevention of Adverse Drug Events
R. Beuscart et al. (Eds.)
IOS Press, 2009

doi:10.3233/978-1-60750-043-8-112

Automatic Indexing in a Drug Information Portal

Saoussen SAKJI[a, b, 1], Catherine LETORD[a], Badisse DAHAMNA[a], Ivan KERGOURLAY[a], Suzanne PEREIRA[a, c], Michel JOUBERT[b] and Stéfan DARMONI[a]
[a] *CISMeF, Rouen University Hospital, Rouen. France & GCSIS, TIBS, LITIS EA 4108, Biomedical Research Institute, Rouen. France*
[b] *LERTIM, EA 3283,Faculty of Medicine, Mediterranean University, Marseille, France*
[c] *Vidal, Issy les Moulineaux, France*

Abstract. *Objective*: The objective of this work is to create a bilingual (French/English) Drug Information Portal (DIP), in a multi-terminological context and to emphasize its exploitation by an ATC automatic indexing allowing having more pertinent information about substances, organs or systems on which drugs act and their therapeutic and chemical characteristics. *Methods*: The development of the DIP was based on the CISMeF portal, which catalogues and indexes the most important and quality-controlled sources of institutional health information in French. DIP has created specific functionalities and uses specific drugs terminologies such as the ATC classification which used to automatic index the DIP resources. *Results*: DIP is the result of collaboration between the CISMeF team and the VIDAL Company, specialized in drug information. DIP is conceived to facilitate the user information retrieval. The ATC automatic indexing provided relevant results in 76% of cases. *Conclusion*: Using multi-terminological context and in the framework of the drug field, indexing drugs with the appropriate codes or/and terms revealed to be very important to have the appropriate information storage and retrieval. The main challenge in the coming year is to increase the accuracy of the approach.

Keywords. Abstracting and indexing as topic, Drug information services, Europe, information storage and retrieval, information, Internet, terminology as subject, vocabulary controlled.

Introduction

Drug information accessible from the Web is plethoric and of very uneven quality. Access to reliable drug information is often difficult for lay people and most of the health professionals without Internet information retrieval skills. Certainly, there are numerous, public or private, on-line drug databases (e.g. PDR [1] and First Databank databases in the US [2] and Vidal database in Europe [3]), which allow to overcome the problem, but their access is often restricted (limited to health professionals, paying, or by registration) and the nature of the information is restricted by national health jurisdictions (Food and Drug Administration in the US [4] and EMEA - European Medicines Agency- in Europe [5]), generating summary of product characteristics (SPC).

[1] Corresponding Author: Sakji.Saoussen@chu-rouen.fr

To resort to an information portal represents a good solution to facilitate the access to reliable and diversified information. Quality-controlled subject portals were defined by Koch [6] as Internet services which apply a comprehensive set of quality measures to support systematic resource discovery. They are defined as Web sites which catalogue the main resources available in a given field, and, generally, they include a search engine. In 2008, the National Library of Medicine (NLM) [7] defined a "drug information portal" which allows querying and reaching information concerning more than 15,000 drugs, stemming from the NLM or from the United States government agencies. The search can be performed by the drug name or by its pharmacological action. To our knowledge, the search by CAS code (Chemical Abstract Service) [8] for chemical substances or by ATC (Anatomical, Therapeutic and Chemical) classification [9] is not possible in this portal.

To go further and to adapt it to the European context, the CISMeF team and the Vidal Company, specialist in drug information, developed a bilingual (French/English) European drug information portal, within the framework of the European project PSIP (Patient Intelligent Safety through Procedures in medication [10]), to respond as much as possible to drug-related questions. The objective of this European Drug Information Portal (DIP) is to describe and index drug quality-resources to improve information retrieval about drugs using multiple terminologies, codes and classifications both international and national.

The objective of this paper is to describe the creation of the specific European Drug Information Portal (DIP), with specific emphasis on its multi-terminological information retrieval. The first exploitation of this portal is done by developing an ATC automatic indexing. An evaluation of this approach is described and the advantages of this indexation on information retrieval, in particular for pharmacists and pharmacologists, are emphasized.

1. Material and Methods

1.1. Description of CISMeF and Description of Health Terminologies

CISMeF (URL: http://www.chu-rouen.fr/cismef) is the French acronym for Catalog and Index of French Language Health Resources on the Internet. It is a health portal which was conceived to catalogue and index the most important and quality-controlled sources of institutional health information in French (N ≈ 64.000), with the aim of providing the most relevant resources to user according to his context [11].

CISMeF uses two standard tools to organize information: the MeSH thesaurus (generally used to index the scientific articles of the MEDLINE bibliographic database) and Dublin Core metadata [12]. The heterogeneity of Internet health resources led the CISMeF team to enhance the MeSH thesaurus, with the introduction of two new concepts: resource types and metaterms. These two new concepts were added to the MeSH descriptors (terms which allow the resource indexing) and the MeSH qualifiers (terms which make it possible to specify the descriptor sense, and to underline one of its particular aspect). CISMeF resource types are an extension of the publication types of MEDLINE and are used to categorize the nature or genre of the content of the resource where MeSH (descriptor/qualifier) pairs describe the topic of the resource. A metaterm is generally a medical specialty or a biological science, which has semantic links with one or more MeSH descriptors, qualifiers and resources types.

To adapt to drug information, CISMeF improved its terminology server: users can access all chemical substances (including drug substances), pharmacological actions, and new resources types related to the drugs. A definition of each one of these resource types was provided either by the CISMeF or the Vidal experts.

Within the MeSH thesaurus, the chemical substance names (including the drug substances) may correspond either to hierarchical MeSH descriptors (N≈25,000) or to MeSH supplementary concept records (SC) (N≈180,000) or synonyms of these terms. The MeSH SCs are terms of reference, not hierarchical, making it possible to describe chemical substances. Without being regarded as descriptors of the MeSH thesaurus, the SCs are semantically related to the latter: on the one hand, for each SC, MeSH recommends a projection towards descriptors; in addition it mentions the descriptor(s) corresponding with the pharmacological(s) action(s) of the described substance, if they exist. In fact, some SCs don't have pharmacological actions. For example, for the SC "cetuximab", MeSH recommends the mapping towards the descriptor "monoclonal antibodies" and specifies that the corresponding pharmacological action is "antineoplastic agents".

With regard to drugs, the most important is to retain the concept of "substance" and not just the concept of supplementary concept or MeSH descriptor. This is why, for the needs of the DIP, we created the concept "Substance" which makes it possible to gather the chemical substances: the MeSH descriptors or the MeSH supplementary concepts. Within the MeSH thesaurus, as within the CISMeF terminology server, the majority of the terms corresponding to substances are connected to pharmacological actions. The substances may have a common pharmacological action.

The development of a terminology adapted to the drugs is also made by the integration of trade (or brand or commercial) names, the International Nonproprietary Names (INN) and of the various national and international codes related to the drugs and chemical substances such as French CIP (Presentation Identifying Code), French CIS (Specialty Identifying Code), French UCD code (Dispensation Common Unit), and the international ATC (Anatomical, Therapeutic and Chemical) code [13] and CAS (Chemical Abstract Service) code [14]. Most of these files were provided to CISMeF by the Vidal Company.

The ATC classification, controlled by the Collaborating Centre for Drug Statistics Methodology of the World Health Organization (WHO), is used to classify the drugs. The drugs are divided into various groups according to the organ or the system on which they act and/or their therapeutic and chemical characteristics. The ATC code has the general form LCCLLCC where (L represents a letter and C a number). In this system, the drugs are classified in five groups at different levels: The 1st level: anatomical group (1 alphabetical character). The 2nd level: principal therapeutic group (2 numerical characters). The 3rd level: therapeutic/pharmacological sub-group (1 alphabetical character). The 4th level: chemical/therapeutic/pharmacological sub-group (1 alphabetical character). The 5th level: sub-group for chemical substance: the individual active ingredient or the association of active ingredients (2 numerical characters). Each level of this classification corresponds to an ATC code and an ATC label. The label of the 5th level corresponds to the International Nonproprietary Name of the substance, when it exists. This code is allocated according to its principal indication. However, the latter can vary from one country to another, which explains why there can be several ATC codes for the same drug according to the country concerned. Approximately 10% of the drugs do not have the same ATC code between France and Denmark (internal study carried out by the Vidal Company for project

PSIP). It was thus necessary for us to adapt to the French and Danish context to overcome with the problem of the varying ATC.

The CAS registry number of polymeric chemicals, a biological sequence or an alloy corresponds to its unique recording number in the Chemical Abstract Service database (CAS), a division of American Chemical Society (ACS). The CAS assigns these numbers, identifiable by an algorithm. Within the MeSH thesaurus, the CAS codes are connected to the MeSH descriptors and the MeSH SCs, which correspond to substances and thus were integrated into the CISMeF terminology server.

In France, the CIS includes 8 digits and is allocated to the pharmaceutical specialties being or having made the subject of a drug approval. It is managed in France by the AFSSAPS (French acronym for French Agency of sanitary security of health products) and in European Union by the EMEA (European Medicines Evaluation Agency). The CIP (code with 7 digits and more recently with 13 digits) identifies the presentation of a pharmaceutical specialty. It is also managed by the French AFSSAPS. A drug can be identified by several CIS numbers, which refer to a different dosage and/or a different dosage form for a specific drug. For the same CIS code, we can have several CIP codes according to the various existing presentations (size and/or conditioning). The UCD code (Common Unit of Dispensation), characterizes the smallest unit used for the drugs dispensation in the care establishments. The UCD code is formed by 7 digits established by the Club Inter Pharmaceutical, and published in the French Official Journal.

1.2. Methodology to Build the Drug Information Portal

The construction of the Drug Information Portal (URL: http://doccismef.chu-rouen.fr/servlets/DIP) is drawn on the CISMeF portal, of which it is a component with specific functionalities. For industrial protection reasons, this site is protected by an identifier and a password. Currently, DIP in Europe gives access to 24,913 resources in French and 837 resources in bilingual (French/English) language. DIP was developed in four steps:

1.2.1. Creation of the Metaterm "Drug"

The CISMeF team has created a metaterm "drug" and has manually attached to it all the MeSH descriptors in relation with drug such as: *pharmacological actions*, *drug marketing authorization* and *drug contamination*. Then, we selected the qualifiers which are used to index the documents concerning drugs namely: *drug action and chemical substances*, *pharmacokinetics*, *drug therapy* and *administration and dosage*. Lastly, we bound to this metaterm all the documents which had been described with the resource type *drug information* and implicitly all the hierarchically lower resource types : *drug evaluation*, *evaluation of the transparency committee*, *guidelines for drug use*, *monograph pharmacy*, *package leaflet*, *pharmacovigilance note*, *summary of product characteristics*. The regrouping of these terms on the level of the metaterm "drug" makes it possible to join together all the documents related to the drug.

1.2.2. Creation of the Portal Site

DIP contains primarily search tools inspired largely by the Doc'CISMeF search engine, but with some specificities focused on drugs. The DIP search tools contain a bilingual (French and English) simple and advanced search. These two search modes are specific of a country (France or Denmark for example), because of the varying ATC codes for the same drug, according to the country.

Simple search can be done by the generic or brand name or the INN, or by any code related to drugs. Advanced search allows a specific search by all the elements describing the drugs: generic name/Brand name, INN (International Nonproprietary Name), pharmacological action, ATC code, CAS number and CIP code, CIS code and UCD code (only French form).

Thus, a search can be conducted in different manners thanks to these various codes. These various accesses are devoted to various users (physicians, pharmacists, pharmacologists, toxicologists), for this reason it was necessary to adapt the search forms according to the needs of the user.

Moreover, the same drug active ingredient can have several ATC codes according to the recognized indications, it was thus necessary to adapt to the French context and the Danish context to solve the problem of the varying ATC. This adaptation was made possible thanks to the participation of the Vidal Company, which provided the adequate files.

1.2.3. Creation of the Contextual Links

The third step allows the implementation of the contextual links towards English speaking data and information bases in particular Drug Information Portal of the US National Library of Medicine (NLM) [15], and search tools of the National Center for Biotechnology Information (NCBI, NLM and NIH) in health sciences, which includes in particular Pub Med/MEDLINE and the NIH chemical databases. These contextual links are based on the translation of French MeSH terms to English MeSH terms.

1.2.4. Development of the "Google selection DIP"

Lastly, we created a specific Google drug search, named "Google selection DIP", making it possible to carry out Google searches limited to a selection of health quality-controlled web sites relating to drugs and previously selected by the CISMeF team. We used "Google™ Custom Search Engine" (Google CSE), by using the platform "Google Co-op™" [16]. It is possible to define a customized version of Google, based on the search engine Google. We provided to Google a list of quality sites editors, already listed by CISMeF but limited to the field of the drug (N=79), to create Google-DIP. These editor sites are the most important French institutional sites (like the High Health Authority or the National Drug Safety Agency). As the Google crawler covers at least all the static pages of a site, the corpus of Google DIP should include all the resources of DIP, but also the other pages which were not selected manually by the CISMeF team. For the Danish version of the DIP, a specific list will have to be defined by the Danish partners of the project PSIP. The query results in the DIP are presented as descriptive notes giving directly access to information emanating not only from French speaking or European institutions (like the EMEA), but also from medical societies.

1.3. Methodology to Index DIP Resources

To exploit the DIP and to improve the description of its resources about drugs, the CISMeF team has chosen the ATC classification as the second controlled vocabulary, besides the MeSH thesaurus and team has decided to restrict as much as possible ATC automatic indexing to DIP resources dealing with a unique substance or association of substances with a unique ATC code. To do so, we have restricted the DIP corpus (n=24,913) to resources having the resources types *drug information* and those which subsume it (n=10,250) (see step1). In the framework of the ATC automatic indexing approach, three subsequent methods of indexation by ATC code were defined (see Figure1):

- Method by title: the search for the ATC code in the resource title.
- Method by brand name: the search for the brand name in the resource title and the allocation of the corresponding ATC code.
- Method by indexation: the search for the ATC code according to the resource indexation (indexation by descriptors and/or SCs).

To set up this strategy, some pre-processing was needed. For that purpose, the ATC codes were automatically mapped with MeSH descriptors, on the one hand, and with the SCs on the other hand. This allows putting into relation the ATC terms and the substances (MeSH descriptors/ SCs), in order to extend the ATC classification system with indexation terms. To do it, usual Natural Language Processing techniques of mapping were used (separation of words, removal of stop words, stemming, terms mapping). Then, the results were validated by a human expert to resolve some missing errors not detectable automatically (e.g. add the MeSH descriptor *potassium compounds* if the term *potassium* is present in the ATC wording, the MeSH descriptor *drug combinations* if the term "association" is present in the ATC wording, or if the ATC wording represents an association of some substances). Moreover, the mapping module must support the explosion of several MeSH descriptors. For example, the ATC term *dexamethasone and antiinfective* having as code *S01CA01* must be mapped with either, the MeSH descriptors *anti-infective agents*, *drug combinations* and *dexamethasone*, or with the MeSH descriptors *drug combinations*, *dexamethasone* and all the MeSH descriptors which subsume the MeSH descriptor *anti-infective agents.* Therefore, thanks to the previous mapping, the ATC term *dexamethasone and antiinfective* is mapped with the MeSH descriptors *drug combinations*, *dexamethasone* and *anti-infective agents, urinary* since the MeSH descriptor *anti-infective agents, urinary* is hierarchical under the MeSH descriptor *anti-infective agents.*

1st step*:* Automatic detection of the ATC 5th level code, including seven characters, in the resource title. If the detection is positive, the ATC code is allocated to the resource and its ATC hierarchical arborescence, mainly for teaching purpose, will be displayed when the resource is queried (Figure 2).

Otherwise, 2nd step*:* Automatic detection of the brand name in the resource title. If the detection is positive, the ATC code associated to this brand name is allocated to the resource. The correlation between the brand name and ATC codes is partially provided by the Hospital Information System of Rouen.

If no results, 3rd step*:* Automatic detection of the ATC code corresponding to the resource due to the indexation terms (MeSH descriptors and/or MeSH SCs) of the resource. In fact, due to the relation between descriptors MeSH and ATC wording and SCs and ATC wording, it is possible to determine the ATC code of the resource indexed by the latter. At this step, as a resource can be indexed by several descriptors and/or SCs, we can obtain as a result several ATC codes. To mitigate this confusion, a score is attributed to every returned ATC code. This score quantifies the link between the ATC codes and the terms of indexation. A score of an ATC code is higher if more terms (MeSH descriptors and/or SCs) are mapped to this ATC code.

During this 3rd step, rules of post-coordination are used. In fact, to manage the automatic ATC indexing of drugs associations, the resource should be indexed by an ATC code if and only if all the terms (MeSH descriptors and SCs) resulted from the mapping module are present in the resource indexation. A check up module verifies that every ATC code found is mapped with all indexation terms which are previously mapped. For example, a resource should be indexed by the ATC code *S01CA01,* if and only if the resource is indexed by all the MeSH descriptors *anti-infective agents*, *drug combinations* and *dexamethasone.*

For every SC, the MeSH recommends a projection towards MeSH descriptors. In this case, the resource should be indexed only by the ATC code which is mapped with the SC because it is considered more pertinent. For example, the MeSH recommends using the MeSH descriptor *azepines* for the SC *cetiedil.* If a resource is indexed with the SC=*cetiedil,* it should be indexed only by the ATC term *cetiedil,* corresponding to the code *C04AX26.* However, this rule is not applicable with the ATC terms which are considered as an association of substances.

At the level of the 2nd step, brand name collision can be detected because several brand names can be mentioned at the resource title. In most cases, these brand names are generic drugs of the same drug with one unique ATC code. In rare cases, these brand names correspond to several ATC codes. Consequently the most suitable ATC code can't be detected.

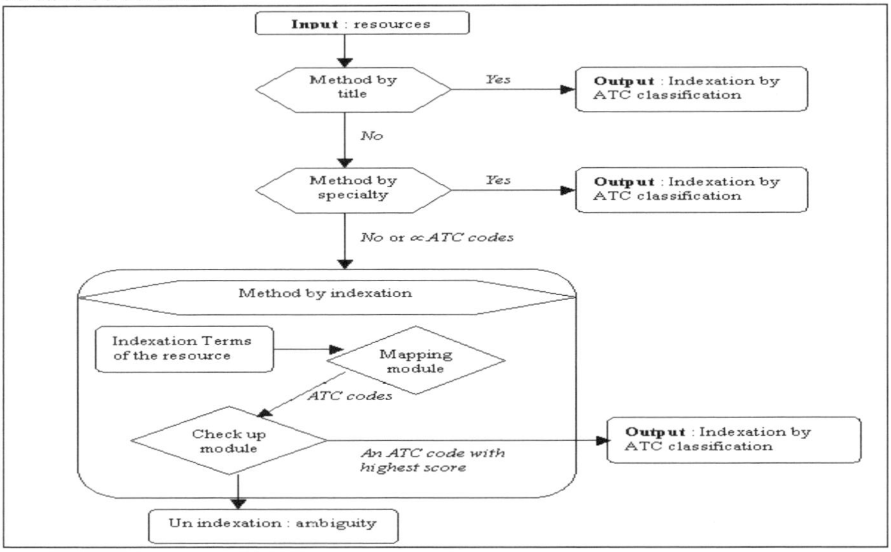

Figure 1. ATC Automatic indexing approach

Test corpus and evaluation: Precision and recall were calculated to show the performance of the automatic mapping between the ATC classification and the MeSH terms (descriptors and SCs), realized during the mapping module. In addition, the performance obtained of the three subsequent methods of ATC automatic indexing is evaluated by the pharmacist expert (CL) who is considered as the gold standard. This evaluation is performed on a DIP corpus with the resources having the resources types: drug information and those which subsume it (n=10,250 out of 24,913; 41.1%): 5,177 MeSH manually indexed resources and 5,073 MeSH automatically indexed resources. From these 10,250 resources, 200 resources were randomly chosen and evaluated by the expert. The qualitative evaluation was rated as: Relevant when the ATC code was correct; Irrelevant when the ATC code was wrong; Partial, when there are potentially several ATC codes and the CISMeF algorithm is displaying only one ATC code, and Incomplete, when the ATC code provided by the algorithm is not providing the complete ATC code including the deepest level (usually the fifth).

2. Results

During the mapping module, the correspondence between the ATC classification and the MeSH terms (descriptors and SCs), was realized in order to find the best matching. The precision was 90% and the recall was 87%. Concerning the three different methods to automatically index ATC (method by title, method by brand name and method by indexation), 3,634 out of 5,073 of MeSH manually indexed resources and 1,341 out of 5,177 of MeSH automatically indexed resources were ATC automatically indexed (see Table 1). Most of the DIP resources are ATC automatically indexed by the method by brand names (51.4% for manually indexed resources and 24.4% for automatically indexed resources), followed by the method by title and the method by indexation.

Table 1. Number of ATC automatic indexed resources according to the type of resources indexation and to the method.

	MeSH Manually indexed resources	MeSH automatically indexed resources
Method by title	722 (14.2%)	0 (0%)
Method by brand name	2608 (51.4%)	1261 (24.4%)
Method by indexation	304 (6.0%)	80 (1.5%)
	3,634 out of 5,073 (71.6%)	1,341 out of 5,177 (25.9%)

Table 2 displays the manual evaluation performed by the pharmacist expert on 200 resources. For these 200 resources (manually and automatically MeSH indexed resources), the overall relevance was 76%, while 20.5% were irrelevant.

Table 2. The manual evaluation of the ATC automatic indexing.

	MeSH manually indexed resources	MeSH automatically indexed resources	Total
Relevant	91 (91%)	61 (61%)	152 (76%)
Irrelevant	5 (5%)	36 (36%)	41 (20.5%)
Partial	3 (3%)	0 (0%)	3 (1.5%)
Incomplete	1 (1%)	3 (3%)	4 (2%)

3. Discussion

To the best of our knowledge, this is the first time that an ATC automatic indexing is applied to a daily operational Web site: Drug Information Portal in Europe.

The performance of the mapping module which provides the correspondence between the ATC classification and the MeSH terms (MeSH descriptors and SCs) in terms of precision and recall is good. The mismatching detected is mainly due to:

- Many several SCs which are not translated in French [2] and some ATC

[2] the SCs are translated in French progressively by the pharmacist expert

wordings without any MeSH equivalent.

- The mapping between an ATC code and SCs is privileged to a mapping between an ATC code and MeSH descriptor(s). For example, the ATC code *J07CA02* having the wording *Diphtheria-pertussis-poliomyelitis-tetanus* was automatically mapped to the MeSH descriptors *whooping cough, diphtheria, poliomyelitis, tetanus* and *drug combinations*, instead of the SC *DTPP vaccine*.

The validation and the error corrections were performed by the pharmacist expert.

The ATC automatic indexing is mainly performed by the method by brand name. This is due to the fact that the ATC automatic indexing is applied on the DIP with resources types "drug information" and those which subsume it, so the brand names of drugs are often mentioned in the resource title.

The null result of ATC automatic indexing by the method by title is due to the CISMeF editorial policy according to which every resource coming from European and French institutions (e.g. EMEA) should be manually indexed with MeSH thesaurus. The resources having an ATC code in the title (added by the CISMeF librarian) are edited by theses European and French institutions.

Overall, for the 200 evaluated resources, the relevance was 76%, while irrelevance was 20.5%. To illustrate irrelevant results, for example, a resource was indexed by the "method by brand name" with the ATC code *G04BE03*: *sildenafil*. However, even the resource title is "Revatio-sildenafil", in this document, the drug is used for treating the lung arterial high blood pressure, and not the erectile dysfunction. So the indexation should be with the ATC term *C04AX: Other peripheral vasodilators* and not the ATC term *G04BE03*: *sildenafil* belonging to the ATC hierarchy *G04BE: Drugs used in erectile dysfunction*

Partial results appeared when there are potentially several ATC codes and the CISMeF algorithm is displaying only one ATC code: e.g. the brand name *thiovalone* has two ATC codes *R02AA05* and *R01AD07*, whereas a single ATC code is detected by the algorithm. Incomplete results appeared when the ATC code provided by the algorithm is not the complete ATC code including the deepest level: e.g. the ATC code *J07BH* is detected instead the ATC code *J07BH02*.

Figure 2 illustrates a spelling error: even if the ATC code is present in the title, the resource indexation was performed thanks to the third method by indexation. The ATC code was not detected at the first step of the approach due to its wrong spelling (L01A X03).

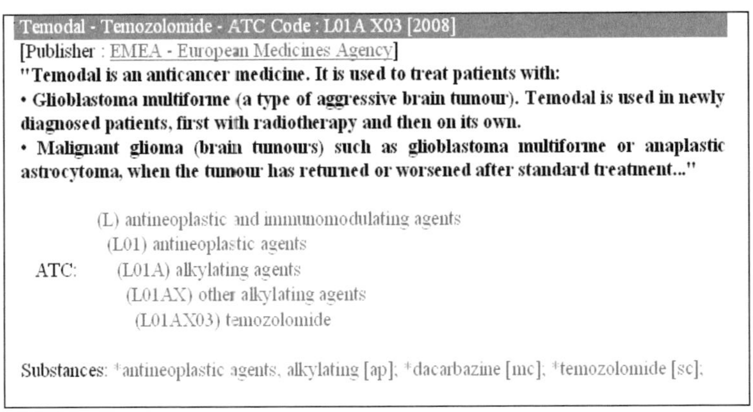

Figure 2. ATC automatic indexing

For educational purposes, instead of displaying the ATC leaf level (usually the fifth), the CISMeF team has decided to display all the ATC hierarchy (Figure 2) to contextualize as much as possible drug information and to supply more information concerning the ATC classification system and consequently improve knowledge about drugs. End-users, and in particular medical students, may obtain information about drugs, the organs or the systems on which they act and their therapeutic and chemical characteristics. A formal evaluation will be needed to prove the accuracy of this editorial choice.

In March 2009, the Vidal Company has provided updated versions of tables ATC-brand names and ATC-INN (MeSH descriptors or SCs), which should improve the results of this ATC automatic indexing. The collaboration with the Vidal Company may lead in the near future to a multi-lingual Drug Information Portal: it needs the addition of European brand names and the translation of the various terminologies (MeSH, ATC) in various European languages. The Vidal Company planned an integration of the current PSIP DIP in several of its commercial products during the third quarter of 2009.

In 2008, the NLM set up the "NLM Drug Information Portal". This portal gives access to information concerning more than 12,000 drugs. Search can also be made with the generic name or the trade name. To our knowledge, research by CAS code or ATC code is not yet possible in this US Drug Information Portal, while CAS number search is possible in PubMed. The development of an advanced search form in the PSIP DIP makes it also possible to better refine the search, crossing, for example, an INN with a pharmacological action. The results underscore the need for a basic understanding of the substances characteristics; effective use of chemical dictionary files; awareness of indexing by codes; and a well-planned search strategy that includes flexibility to make changes as necessary in order to complete a successful search.

The Health French Ministry is planning to design a Governmental Drug Information Portal in 2009, where the content has to be limited to french government sources. The current PSIP DIP is sufficiently scalable to answer to this reduced content compared to the current content described in this paper.

4. Conclusion

In this paper, we have described a specific drug information portal, with specific emphasis on its multi-terminological (in particular, MeSH thesaurus, ATC classification) information retrieval. To our knowledge, this approach is quite innovative.

Acknowledgments

This work was partially granted by the PSIP project (Patient Safety through Intelligent Procedures in medication, 7th Framework Program of the European Union, Grant agreement n° 216130).

References

[1] The Physicians' Desk Reference web site URL: http://www.pdr.net/login/Login.aspx [accessed 2009 April09].
[2] The First DataBank URL: http://www.firstdatabank.com/ [accessed 2009 April09].
[3] Leading information about the health products. URL: http://www.vidal.fr/fiches-medicaments [accessed 2009 April09].
[4] Center for Drug Evaluation and Research. The Food and Drug Administration URL: http://www.accessdata.fda.gov/Scripts/cder/DrugsatFDA/ [accessed 2009 April09].
[5] European Medicines Agency URL: http://www.emea.europa.eu/ [accessed 2009 April09].
[6] T. Koch, Quality-controlled subject gateways: definitions, typologies, empirical overview, Subject gateways. Online Information Review (2000), 24-34.
[7] US NLM Drug Information Portal; URL: http://druginfo.nlm.nih.gov/drugportal/drugportal.jsp [accessed 2009 April09].
[8] P.G. Dittmar, R.E. Stobaugh, C.E. Watson, The Chemical Abstracts Service Chemical Registry System. I. General Design. Journal of Chemical Information and Computer Sciences, vol. 16, no. 2, 111, 1976
[9] A. Skrbo, B. Begović, S. Skrbo, Classification of drugs using the ATC system (Anatomic, Therapeutic, Chemical Classification) and the latest changes. Med Arh (2004), 138-41.
[10] PSIP (Patient Safety through Intelligent Procedures in medication). URL: www.psip-project.eu [accessed 2009 April09].
[11] S.J. Darmoni, E. Amsallem, M. Haugh, B. Lukacs, V. Leroux, B. Thirion, J. Weber, J.P. Boissel, Level of evidence as a future gold standard for the content quality of health resources on the internet. Methods Inf Med 42 (2003), 220-5.
[12] M. Dekkers, S. Weibel. State of the Dublin Core Metadata Initiative. D-Lib Magazine, vol. 9, no. 4, 2003. URL: http://webdoc.sub.gwdg.de/edoc/aw/d-lib/dlib/april03/weibel/04weibel.html [accessed 2009 April09].
[13] A. Skrbo B. Begović S. Skrbo. "Classification of drugs using the ATC system (Anatomic, Therapeutic, Chemical Classification) and the latest changes," Med Arh. Vol. 58(1 Suppl 2), 138-141, 2004. Bosnian. PMID: 5137231
[14] P.G. Dittmar, R.E. Stobaugh, C.E. Watson. "The Chemical Abstracts Service Chemical Registry System. I. General Design." Journal of Chemical Information and Computer Sciences, vol. 16, no. 2, 111, 1976.
[15] US NLM Drug Information Portal; URL: http://druginfo.nlm.nih.gov/drugportal/drugportal.jsp [accessed 2009 April09].
[16] Google Coop; URL: http://www.google.com/coop/ [accessed 2009 April09].

Detection and Prevention of Adverse Drug Events
R. Beuscart et al. (Eds.)
IOS Press, 2009

doi:10.3233/978-1-60750-043-8-123

Implementation of SNOMED CT to the Medicines Database of a General Hospital

Francisco J. FARFÁN SEDANO [a], Marta TERRÓN CUADRADO [a, 1], Eva M. GARCÍA REBOLLEDO [a], Yolanda CASTELLANOS CLEMENTE [a], Pablo SERRANO BALAZOTE [b], Ángel GÓMEZ DELGADO [b]

[a]Pharmacy Department
[b]MedicalDirector
Hospital Universitario de Fuenlabrada. Camino del Molino, 2. 28009-Fuenlabrada. Madrid. España

Abstract. A concept-based terminology that covers all features of healthcare is essential for the development of an Electronic Health Record (EHR). Since a significant percentage of the EHR can be drug related information, we decided to implement the controlled drug terminology provided by SNOMED CT to achieve the potential benefit to promote Patient Safety that a fully functional pharmacy system can offer. One of the expected advantages of our Project is to establish a bridge between reference terminology and the drug knowledge databases. There is also an economic advantage of implementing a "clinical drug product", the one defined by the drug name, its strength and dose form, instead of the manufactured drug product. The Pharmacy economic management of stocks and response to the offers from the pharmaceutical companies is another expected asset of the Project. This Project is intended as well to give support to a more widespread objective of interoperability with the Primary Care systems.

Keywords. Patient Safety, SNOMED CT, terminology, semantic interoperability, medicines.

Introduction

After the released in 1999 of the United States Institute of Medicine (IOM) report *To Err is Human: Building a Safer Health System*, international attention has focused on the potential risks that patients undergo when they receive medical treatment [1]. That report noted that as many as 98,000 people die each year as a result of medical errors, 7,000 from medication errors alone. The influence of the IOM report has been enormous and captured widespread media coverage and stimulated renewed professional and public dialogue about patient safety.

Adverse drug events, as previously mentioned, are among the most dangerous side-effects of medical treatment. In the Netherlands over 5% of all emergency admissions are related to adverse drug events, 4% in the United Kingdom. The risk of such an adverse event occurring in a hospital is considerably higher [2] [3] [4] [5].

A new IOM report released in July 2006, *Preventing Medication Errors* [6], agrees that we still have much work to do. The report calls the frequency of medication errors

[1] Corresponding Author: mterron.hflr@salud.madrid.org

and related injuries "a serious concern" and suggests numerous error-preventing strategies that will require health care professionals attention, including electronic prescribing, improved pharmacy leaflets and medication-related information on the Internet for consumers, better communication of patient information to those who need it, and collaboration among industry, FDA, and patient safety organizations to address problems with drug naming, labelling and packaging.

When analysing the traditional components of medication use and where medication errors occur, Leape and cols. in their renowned study published in 1995 found that 39% of errors occurred during the prescribing phase, 12% during transcription, 11% during dispensing, and 38% during administration. Consequently, much emphasis has been placed on the use of technology in prescribing. There are good reasons for this, including the many errors that involve misinterpreted handwriting or errors-prone abbreviations, the prescribing of inappropriate doses, and the occurrence of interactions and allergic reactions. Eliminating handwritten orders and implementing medication-checking software with decision support in prescribing systems can prevent such errors. However, the goal of every health care organisation should be to incorporate technology across the whole medication management spectrum.

Acknowledging that concern about patient safety, around the world, there is an increasing recognition that electronic health records (EHR) can foster improvement in health outcomes and in the efficiency of Health Services.

Although to fully realise the potential of EHR systems, a timely and secure access to such systems needs to be ensured to all health care professionals that are entitled to use them. Moreover, the information contained in EHRs should be up-to-date, accurate and, in its communication to another location, system or language should be correctly understood. This is called interoperability. Interoperable EHR systems are certainly enabling tools to promote patient centred care, a lifeline for continuity of care and support to mobility of patients.

However, the development of Information and Communication Technologies (ICT) systems and services has resulted in a proliferation of incompatible ICT formats and standards in healthcare institutions. The resulting lack of interoperability (the ability to "talk to each other") between health ICT systems in different regions and countries causes problems when patients travel or simply when admitted or discharged from Hospital in his own country of origin. The deployment of interoperable systems will support the free movement of people and services and will favour the safety of travelling individuals.

Interoperable EHR systems and services do not necessarily lead to harmonisation of national or local/regional healthcare systems; nevertheless, they are a key element in working towards harmonisation of essential medical information and the accessibility of this information to provide patients with more effective and efficient healthcare, by having timely and secure access to basic, and possibly vital, healthcare information.

To progress on interoperability across different Health Care Providers the core applications that have been described at European and international level are patient summary and electronic prescribing. In this strategy the most challenging part is to achieve semantic interoperability of EHR systems. Semantic interoperability has been defined as ensuring that the precise meaning of exchanged information is understandable by any other system or application not initially developed for this purpose.

In the purpose of achieving interoperable EHR systems we need to represent the relevant health information through data structures (such as archetypes and templates), and subsets of terminology systems and ontologies responsive to local user needs. SNOMED CT is one of the terminologies that could help in this objective [7].

1. Objective

The objective of this Project is to implement the controlled terminology of SNOMED CT to the medicines database of the Pharmacy Department system and, simultaneously, to the medicines database of the Hospital EHR system with the final aim of creating a knowledge-based model for medicines in benefit of the patient.

2. Methods

2.1. The Terminology SNOMED CT

SNOMED CT is a comprehensive clinical terminology that provides clinical content and expressivity for clinical documentation and reporting [8]. It can be used to code, retrieve, and analyse clinical data. It represents a major step towards providing that common reference terminology which is essential for the EHR and for the improvement of patient safety.

SNOMED CT resulted from the merge of SNOMED Reference Terminology developed by the College of American Pathologists and Clinical Terms Version 3 developed by the National Health Service of the United Kingdom.

The controlled terminology provided by SNOMED CT represents the whole scope of clinical information about patients organised in different hierarchies:

Table 1. Top-level Hierarchies in SNOMED CT

Clinical finding
Procedure
Observable entity
Body structure
Organism
Substance
Pharmaceutical/biological
Specimen
Special concept
Physical object
Physical force
Event
Environments/ geographical locations
Social context
Situation with explicit context
Staging and scales
Linkage concept
Qualifier value
Record artefact

Convinced of the importance of a standardised clinical terminology to foster the safe exchange of clinical information, nine countries joined together in March 2007 to launch the International Health Terminology Standards Development Organisation

(IHTSDO). Subsequently, that organisation negotiated the purchase and support of SNOMED CT, committing itself to broaden the use of SNOMED CT, within and across countries and professions, accelerate progress on terminology development and maintenance, and strengthen the Community of Practice and the tools to support it.

The basic components of SNOMED CT are *concepts*, *descriptions* and *relationships*. A concept is a clinical meaning identified by a unique numerical identifier (ConceptID) that never changes. Concepts are represented by a unique human-readable Fully Specified Name (FSN). Concepts are formally defined in terms of their relationships with other concepts, the advantage of which is that these logical definitions give explicit meaning which a computer can process and query on. In addition, every concept has also a set of terms that name the concept in a human-readable way.

Concepts in SNOMED CT can be very general or represent increasingly specific levels of detail (granularity) improving the capability to code clinical data at the appropriate level of detail.

In SNOMED CT each concept has a unique numerical identifier, ConceptID, which do not have hierarchical or implicit meaning. That numerical identifier does not reveal any information about the nature of the concept.

Additionally, there are concept descriptions, different terms assigned to a SNOMED CT concept. Multiple descriptions might be associated with a concept identified with its ConceptID. For example, *myocardial infarction* is associated with the following synonyms *cardiac infarction*, *heart attack*, and *infarction of heart*.

From 1996 there is a Spanish edition of SNOMED CT [9] developed by a team of translators based in Buenos Aires, Argentina, working collaboratively with the College of American Pathologists and medical professionals from other countries. Also in Buenos Aires, the Hospital Italiano has implemented an advanced terminology service based in SNOMED CT [10] [11] [12] whose primary objective was to homogenize data collection. Although, the final aim of the project has wider relevance, to lay the foundations for future clinical decision support systems. Particularly, the Medical Informatics Department has implemented SNOMED CT to the Argentinean pharmaceutical products.

2.2. The Hospital Universitario de Fuenlabrada

The Hospital Universitario de Fuenlabrada is a public general hospital located in the Madrid Region which started its activity in 2004 to provide care assistance to a population of 217.000 inhabitants. From the begining the Hospital Universitario de Fuenlabrada implemented an EHR system highly integrated with the Primary Care EHR system and the specific computer applications from different providers installed in the Pharmacy and other Departments.

The Hospital strategy has been therefore to integrate distributed data resources. The standard HL7 was chosen to enable the integration of the EHR system (SELENE) and the Pharmacy application (FarmaTools) which manages all the activity related to drug therapy in the Hospital. It implies treatments administered in clinical wards (in-patient bed areas), out-patients, and Day Hospital (the specific area within the Hospital which provides services for specific therapies namely oncological protocols).

Internationally, efforts have been made in the area of medical informatics to forge a single, standardized, multipurpose terminology or terminology model for representing medication. However, much of the work is still in progress and a common terminology for drugs is the goal of different organisations.

Coding schemes at international level include the National Drug Codes (NDC codes), RxNorm, and the Anatomic Therapeutic Chemical (ATC) Index [13] [14] [15]. In addition, several commercial drug knowledge base vendors provide comprehensive drug databases, product-specific drug information as well as other encoded knowledge that support clinical functions relevant to drug therapy. These drug databases are designed to support specific pharmacy applications but do not necessarily fit the model for a controlled vocabulary.

Our objective was in that scenario to implement the controlled drug terminology provided by SNOMED CT with the aim of achieving the support to a number of functions within healthcare to promote patient safety:

- Electronic prescribing
- Recording medication histories within electronic patient records
- Electronic transfer of medication histories between diverse systems
- Interaction with clinical decision support systems (e.g. drug-drug interactions, allergy alerts, range for drug dosing, …)
- Aid clinical audit and quality assurance activities
- Aggregation of drug prescribing and dispensing information for analysis
- Assist in healthcare research

As previously mentioned, SNOMED CT is organized into hierarchies. In our Project we implemented the ConceptID and descriptions of medicines included in the *Pharmaceutical/ biological product hierarchy.*

In SNOMED CT this hierarchy was introduced as a top-level hierarchy in order to clearly distinguish drug products (products) from their chemical constituents (substances). It contains concepts that represent the multiple levels of granularity required to give support to different use cases such as computerized physician order entry (CPOE) or e-prescribing, decision support tools and formulary management. Different levels of granularity are needed depending on the desired functionality. For a system to alert drug-drug interactions, specificity down to the ingredient level is essential, where as for prescribing purposes, additional levels of granularity are required.

We focused our efforts on the most granular level, the *"virtual medicinal product"* in SNOMED CT. We chose that concept because it represents the **clinical drug** that physicians prescribe and nurses administer to the patient, that is to say, **ingredient, strength and dose form.** This information is contained in the Fully Specified Name description of SNOMED CT. For example, a clinical drug would be *clonazepam 2mg tablet* (Figure 1).

Consequently, to implement the terminology of SNOMED CT and restructure our database to a clinical drug product concept is the goal of our Project. Instead of using the manufactured drug product name, the clinical drug would be the core item of our database. From the economic point or view, this clinical drug will gather different manufactured products with the same component, the same strength, and dose form produced by the diverse pharmaceuticals companies. That approach allows the Pharmacy Department logistics to easily purchase the best option available.

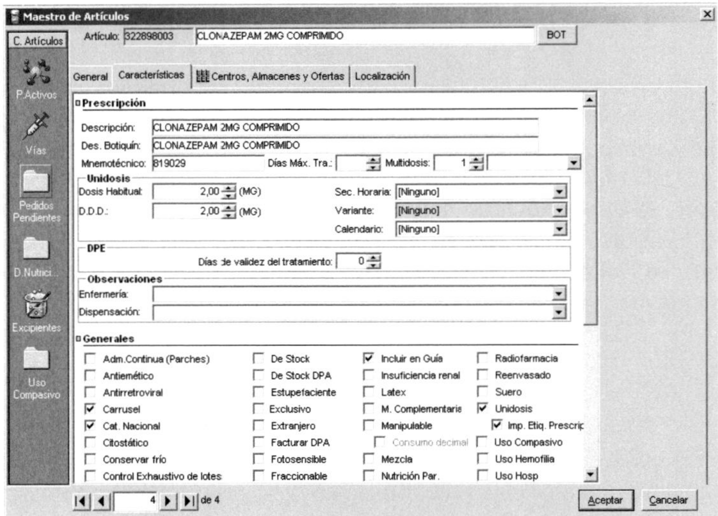

Figure 1. Medicines database (Pharmacy informatics system)

The integration of the Pharmacy system with the patient's EHR system, which contains the physician's prescription, requires adapting simultaneously both databases (Figure 2).

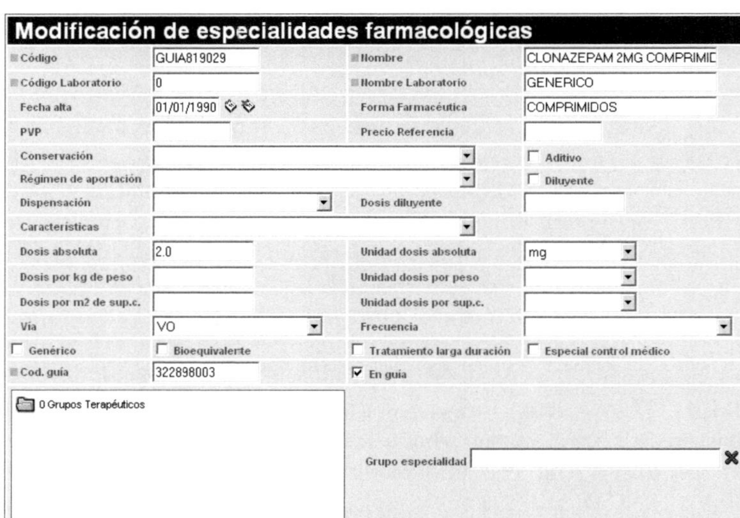

Figure 2. Medicines database (Electronic Health Record system)

3. Results

To date, we have implemented 700 clinical drug products in our database according to the SNOMED CT terminology. Simultaneously, the medicines database contained in the Hospital EHR system has been changed to enable the integration between both systems.

A significant percentage of the existing commercial drug products in Spain are not represented at the present edition of SNOMED CT. To date, we have been unable to obtain the corresponding ConceptID and description for 200 Spanish manufactured products, 22% of the clinical drugs searched. This situation reflects the different pharmaceutical markets in Europe and in the United States.

Each clinical drug gathers the commercially available products manufactured by the pharmaceutical companies allowing the Pharmacy Department to respond rapidly to the economic proposals received.

4. Discussion

The implementation of a concept-based terminology to the medicines database of our Hospital enables us to build the fundamentals of a knowledge-based model for medicines in benefit of the patient.

To complete our Project we need extensions, modifications to the released version of SNOMED CT, due to the lack of clinical drug products not represented at this moment. The SNOMED CT technical structure allows that extensibility to new concepts ensuring the current features of consistency and interoperability.

References

[1] Kohn LT, Corrigan JM, Donaldson MS, editors. To err is human: Building a safer health system. Committee on Health Care in America. Institute of Medicine. Washington (DC): National Academy Press; 1999.

[2] Otero MJ, Alonso P, Martín R, et al. Analysis of preventable adverse drug events (ADEs) leading to hospital admission: incidence, categorization and cost. 36th ASHP Midyear Clinical Meeting and Exhibits, December 2-6,2001 New Orleans, LA.

[3] López Y, Otero MJ, Alonso P, et al. Estudio prospectivo de los acontecimientos adversos por medicamentos (AAM) en pacientes hospitalizados. Rev Clin Esp 2000; 200:106.

[4] Martín MT, Codina C, Tuset M, et al. Problemas relacionados con la medicación como causa del ingreso hospitalario. Med Clin (Barc) 2002; 118: 205-10.

[5] Veli N. Stroetmann, Jean-Pierre Thierry, Karl A. Stroetmann, Alexander Dobrev. eHealth for Safety-Impact of ICT on Patient Safety and Risk Management. Office for Official Publications of the European Communities. Luxembourg; 2007.

[6] Committee on Health Care in America. Institute of Medicine. Preventing Medication errors. Washington (DC): National Academy Press; 2006.

[7] Rector AL. Barriers, approaches and research priorities for integrating biomedical ontologies. SemanticHEALTH (2008).

[8] The International Health Terminology Standards Development Organization. SNOMED CLINICAL TERMS User Guide. January 2007 Release.

[9] Reynoso GA, March AD, Berra CM, Strobietto RP, Barani M, Iubatti M, Chiaradio MP, Serebrisky D, Kahn A, Vaccarezza OA, Leguiza JL, Ceitlin M, Luna DA, Bernaldo de Quirós FG, Otegui MI, Puga MC, Vallejos M. Development of the Spanish version of the Systematizad Nomenclature of Medicine: methodology and main issues. Proc AMIA Symp. 2000:694-8.

[10] Osornio AL, Luna D, Gambarte ML, Gómez A, Reynoso G, de Quirós FG. Creation of a local interface terminology to SNOMED CT. Stud Health Technol Inform. 2007; 129 (Pt 1):765-9.

[11] Navas H, Osornio AL, Baum A, Gómez A, Luna D, de Quirós FG. Creation and evaluation of a terminology server for the interactive coding of discharge summaries. Stud Health Technol Inform. 2007; 129 (Pt 1):650-4.

[12] Gambarte ML, Osornio AL, Martínez M, Reynoso G, Luna D, de Quirós FG. A practical approach to advanced terminology services in health information systems. Stud Health Technol Inform. 2007; 129Pt 1):629-5.
[13] The National Drug Code Directory (Food and Drug Administration): http://www.fda.gov/cder/ndc/ Accessed 10/01/2009.
[14] U.S. National Library of Medicine, RxNorm: http://www.nlm.nih.gov/research/umls/rxnorm/index.html Accessed 10/01/2009.
[15] WHO Collaborating centre for Drug Statistics Methodology (WHO): http://www.whocc.no/atcddd/ Accessed 10/01/2009.

Detection and Prevention of Adverse Drug Events
R. Beuscart et al. (Eds.)
IOS Press, 2009

doi:10.3233/978-1-60750-043-8-131

A Knowledge Engineering Framework towards Clinical Support for Adverse Drug Event Prevention: The PSIP Approach

Vassilis KOUTKIAS [a], George STALIDIS [a], Ioanna CHOUVARDA [a], Katerina LAZOU [a], Vassilis KILINTZIS [a] and Nicos MAGLAVERAS [a, 1]
[a] *Aristotle University, Medical School, Lab of Medical Informatics, Thessaloniki, GREECE*

Abstract. Adverse Drug Events (ADEs) are currently considered as a major public health issue, endangering patients' safety and causing significant healthcare costs. Several research efforts are currently concentrating on the reduction of preventable ADEs by employing Information Technology (IT) solutions, which aim to provide healthcare professionals and patients with relevant knowledge and decision support tools. In this context, we present a knowledge engineering approach towards the construction of a Knowledge-based System (KBS) regarded as the core part of a CDSS (Clinical Decision Support System) for ADE prevention, all developed in the context of the EU-funded research project PSIP (Patient Safety through Intelligent Procedures in Medication). In the current paper, we present the knowledge sources considered in PSIP and the implications they pose to knowledge engineering, the methodological approach followed, as well as the components defining the knowledge engineering framework based on relevant state-of-the-art technologies and representation formalisms.

Keywords. Adverse Drug Events, Knowledge Engineering, Knowledge-based System, Ontologies, Rules, Guideline Modelling, Clinical Decision Support

Introduction

Nowadays, Adverse Drug Events (ADEs) due to medication errors and human factors constitute a major public health issue, endangering patients' safety and causing significant healthcare costs. Information Technology (IT) is envisioned to play an important role towards the reduction of preventable ADEs by providing healthcare professionals and patients with relevant knowledge and decision support tools [1].

In this work, we present a knowledge engineering approach towards the construction of a Knowledge-based System (KBS) regarded as the core part of a CDSS (Clinical Decision Support System) for ADE prevention. The CDSS that is aimed at providing support in everyday clinical practice for the prevention of drug-related errors is under development within the EU-funded project PSIP (Patient Safety through Intelligent Procedures in Medication). The PSIP project aims at preventing medical

---

[1] Corresponding Author: Nicos Maglaveras, Professor, Lab of Medical Informatics, Medical School, Aristotle University, 54124, P.O. Box 323, Thessaloniki, Greece; Email: nicmag@med.auth.gr.

errors by facilitating the systematic production of knowledge on ADEs and by improving the entire PDAC (Prescribing, Dispensing, Administration and Compliance) cycle in hospital environments. Within the scope of PSIP is to generate a unified model of the ADE-related knowledge extracted from various knowledge sources, which will be consequently used to develop innovative knowledge-based applications. Through knowledge engineering methods, PSIP will deliver professionals and patients a contextualized knowledge framework fitting the local risk parameters in the form of alerts and decision support functions.

In the following, we refer to the knowledge sources considered up to now and the implications they pose to knowledge engineering, as well as on the major parts of the related knowledge engineering requirements. Considering such requirements in conjunction with the state-of-the-art available methodologies, the PSIP knowledge framework was defined and is presented in the following. The purpose of this work is to constitute the initial framework for future implementation of ADE prevention CDSS modules.

1. Rationale and Related Work

Knowledge engineering involves primarily the analysis, construction and maintenance procedures of knowledge, as well as the development of appropriate methods, languages and tools specialized for developing KBSs [2]. Nowadays, there exists an overall consensus that the process of building a KBS may be seen as a modeling activity. Building a KBS corresponds to building a computerized model with the aim of realizing problem-solving capabilities comparable to a domain expert. This modeling view of the building process of a KBS has the following consequences:

- A knowledge model is only an approximation of the reality, and in principle, the modeling process is *infinite*.
- The modeling process is an *iterative* one, as new observations may lead to a refinement, modification or completion of the already built-up model.
- Evaluation is indispensable for the construction of an adequate model, thus the model must be *revisable* in every stage of the modeling process.

In the field of ADE research, the primary focus of IT solutions has been up to now their automatic/semi-automatic identification by employing Machine Learning and statistical inference techniques applied to patient data repositories, e.g. EHRs (Electronic Health Records). Specifically, the aim was to develop techniques that would provide evidence on the origin of ADEs, following typically expert review evaluation of the obtained results. These outcomes were foreseen to constitute the basis for advancing the decision support functionalities offered by Clinical Information Systems (CISs), such as CPOE (Computerized Physician Order Entry) systems, on ADEs; however, the majority of these approaches did not elaborate further towards the incorporation of the ADE patterns/signals identified into actual CDSSs that could provide in turn added value services to CISs in practice. Comprehensive reviews on ADE identification technologies are provided in [1] and [3].

Recently, as more mature evidence on ADE prevalence is gained, the focus of ADE research has also included the incorporation of the ADE patterns/signals identified into sophisticated models that are based on knowledge. For example, in [4] a data mining tool is presented that improves signal detection algorithms by performing terminological reasoning on MedDRA (Medical Dictionary for Regulatory Activities) codes based on Description Logic (DL). The constructed tool implements quantitative techniques based on underlying statistical and Bayesian models, as well as terminological reasoning by employing an inference engine. In continuation of the previous work, the same authors present an ontology constructed for ADE description, in an effort to semantically describe MedDRA terms [5], in order to automatically retrieve and group terms describing similar medical conditions.

In the context of terminological reasoning and ADE management, in [6] a mapping of ADE terms contained in WHO-ART (World Health Organization – Adverse Reaction Terminology) to equivalent SNOMED-CT (Systematized Nomenclature of Medicine - Clinical Terms) concepts contained in the UMLS (Unified Medical Language System) Metathesaurus is proposed. Based on this mapping, the authors automatically classified terms using a DL definition expressing their synonymies. The gold standard in the study was a set of 13 MedDRA special search categories restricted to ADE terms available in WHO-ART.

In [7], a prototype medical intelligent assistant is presented aiming to improve patient care and safety by reducing medical errors in the hospital setting. The system is based on an ontology of hospital care concepts including hospital activities, procedures, and policies, as well as medical knowledge per se. A set of abstract rule types model general situations that need to be identified to detect potential problems and particular instantiations of those rule types identify individual situations. The system is not designed to provide medical diagnosis or support decision making, but rather to track the implications of such medical decisions taken by medical professionals within the context of the guidelines and regulations of the medical environment, and the background of established medical knowledge.

Finally, in [8], the design of a semantically interoperable AE (Adverse Event) reporting framework is presented. The framework consists of the AE ontology, aiming to describe AEs in a semantically interoperable way, and the AE reporting schema to envelope and deliver the content of AE request and report. The ontology was built upon existing AE taxonomies, while the reporting system was designed as a common AE messaging interface in the form of an XML (eXtensible Markup Language) schema. The aim of the proposed AE reporting framework is expected to allow semantic interoperability in sharing and exchange of patient safety information within and among various healthcare information systems.

Typically, the construction of a CDSS based on extended medical knowledge and supporting iterative refinement and contextualisation, as envisioned in PSIP, requires a substantial modelling activity, i.e. deciding what clinical distinctions and data are relevant, identifying the concepts and their relations that bear on the decision-making task, and ascertaining a problem-solving strategy that can use the relevant clinical knowledge to reach appropriate conclusions [9]. Consequently, construction of such a CDSS, entails development of a model encapsulating both the required problem-solving behaviour and the relevant clinical knowledge.

The steps of this modelling procedure as applying to PSIP are described in the following, explaining the rationale behind the adopted approach.

2. Knowledge Sources in PSIP

The knowledge sources considered for ADE identification in PSIP are:

- **ADE rules from data mining**: The outcome of data mining techniques applied on unified patient records originated from the hospitals participating in the project, according to a (specifically designed for analysis) common data structure, that is provided in the form of rules associating the parameters/variables related to ADEs. Data mining initially aimed at detecting atypical hospital stays and, subsequently, at extracting associations among drugs, hospitalisation parameters, patient parameters, diagnoses and observed effects.
- **Drug interactions**: Knowledge on drug-related interactions, e.g. drug to drug, drug to allergy class, drug to contraindications, and so forth, that is already known and registered in existing databases. More specifically, the drug interactions database created and maintained by VIDAL (project partner) was used as primary source for such knowledge.
- **Tacit knowledge**: It is derived from human experts, providing their knowledge and experiences on ADEs.
- **Human factors and clinical procedures**: Constitutes complementary knowledge about factors related to ADEs. These factors are associated with human errors within the context of clinical procedures. The corresponding knowledge could be potentially in the form of electronic guidelines, associating procedures with drugs and conditions.
- **Literature**: Knowledge reported in the literature may be extracted, expressed in an appropriate form (e.g. rules) and imported in the Knowledge Base (KB).

In essence, all the above knowledge sources apart from tacit knowledge encapsulate explicit knowledge that may be expressed via electronic means. While tacit knowledge can not be easily managed and shared, explicit knowledge is typically well articulated and coded, making it rather easily shareable [10]. The knowledge sources from which the PSIP KB will be constructed were analyzed in detail, in order to design a suitable knowledge model, appropriate engineering processes and an effective overall KBS architecture. Issues considered were the format/syntax and possible formalization of each source, the required terminologies, the expected size and complexity, as well as special requirements in expressiveness and processing.

3. Knowledge Engineering Methodologies

In the context of the abovementioned knowledge sources, the major knowledge engineering methodologies that are considered particularly favorable are ontology engineering [11], rule-based systems (RBSs) [12], and electronic guidelines and protocols modeling [13]. These methodologies are envisioned to be complementarily employed to define a single-common knowledge framework for ADE prevention.

In particular, ontology engineering in PSIP is essential towards the construction of the vocabulary/terminology of concepts/variables related to ADEs that take part in the rules originated by the data mining techniques, as well as for the drug interaction rules provided via the VIDAL database. In such an ontology, the appropriate standard terminologies (such as ICD-10, ATC, etc.), according to which the concepts are expressed, have to be incorporated. Additional terms/concepts that are not contained in standard terminologies have to be also defined and encapsulated in the ontology model.

Rule modeling constitutes an important knowledge engineering approach for PSIP, due to the fact that the project elaborates on knowledge discovery for ADEs based on data mining techniques. In particular, the project elaborates on the inference of decision tree induced rules from patient data that are stored in EHRs of the clinical sites participating in the project, as well as on drug interaction rules. Thus, rules have to be effectively represented in the KB and executed by the KBS engine.

Finally, guideline/protocol modeling is particularly important as rules originated from data mining are rather complex, i.e. each rule typically comprises of several intermediate rules; thus, encoding of each rule involves the construction of a conditional workflow, that may be effectively encoded as a guideline/protocol. In addition, guideline/protocol modeling is favorable for representing procedures that are relevant to the PDAC chain currently applied per hospital/department. In this regard, this approach is particularly applicable considering the outcome of the human factors analysis, so as to effectively model the procedure towards ADE avoidance, or providing decision support services in the stages of the procedure that have been identified as the most probable for the occurrence of human errors, with respect to drugs. In general, guideline/protocol modeling enables the unification of domain knowledge (via ontologies) and task/procedural knowledge (e.g. rules) into an efficient problem-solving model that is particularly suited to develop a CDSS.

As the project evolves, new knowledge is expected to be extracted from data mining procedures; thus, new knowledge representation schemes might be potentially required. In this regard, it is evident that knowledge engineering activities will follow an iterative procedure, in order to address potential new requirements concerning knowledge representation.

4. Knowledge Engineering Challenges in PSIP

Knowledge engineering tasks in PSIP aim to create and maintain a KB that is able to store the specific knowledge regarding ADEs that is required by the CDSS, in order to assist in preventing drug-related errors. In this regard, our efforts concentrate on the following major issues:

- knowledge modeling, i.e. necessary formalism, components analysis, concepts and relations definition, identification of constraints, etc.;
- knowledge acquisition, i.e. population of the knowledge model via appropriate tools and APIs (Application Programming Interfaces);
- knowledge verification, in terms of syntax, structure and semantics;
- knowledge management, and
- knowledge querying and inference.

Equally important, the following quality criteria for the knowledge engineering procedure have to be taken into account:

- Reusability of design elements and resulting code,
- maintainability and adaptability (typically, one-step development is usually unrealistic, especially for knowledge-intensive systems),
- ease of knowledge refinements (as knowledge changes over time),
- explanatory power, if possible (which is crucial in medical decision support), and
- contextualization support; for example, each rule is applicable in a particular context, e.g. in a specific hospital, department, country, user type, etc., while features such as confidence, support and percentage of death have to be defined for each context and rule.

As knowledge in PSIP is derived from several sources, a common model is required, suitable for containing all types of knowledge and supporting consolidation mechanisms. The KB will operate in two modes: (a) *learning* or *knowledge capturing mode* (i.e. knowledge encoding and storage), and (b) *access mode* (e.g. offer access to the CDSS). The later will use the knowledge stored in the KB with input parameters (medical context), in order to generate results (e.g. alerts). In addition, a maintenance operation is foreseen including consistency checking and conflict resolution, as well as deletion/revision of obsolete rules. The following specific requirements on the overall approach result from studying the knowledge sources:

- The KB should support a complex model encapsulating rules, ontologies and procedural logic.
- The KB and the CDSS are envisaged as being implemented in one KBS that offers both knowledge management (e.g. editing and storage of knowledge) and decision support (i.e. rule execution in combination with context, in order to produce indications for ADE prevention).
- Although patient data and other context-related information will not be stored in the KB, the vocabulary required to express such data has to be defined in the knowledge model, as the corresponding terms are included in the rules and patient/context information will be used by the CDSS at access mode.
- Protocols, guidelines and/or procedural workflows need to be supported, in order to be able to express effectively the complexity of the rules, as well as knowledge originated from human factor analysis. This requirement is decisive for the selection of the KBS to be adopted in PSIP.

5. Knowledge Framework

The process for knowledge model construction followed in PSIP is based on CommonKADS [14]. This methodology is applicable to a wide range of knowledge engineering applications and can be easily adapted with a number of deviations to individual requirements. The knowledge model construction process can be decomposed in a number of stages, the most significant of which are: a) **Identification**, in which information sources that are useful for knowledge modelling are identified and existing model components (i.e. generic task models and domain-knowledge schemas) are surveyed that could be reused in the project. b) **Specification**, involving the specifications of the knowledge model that are expressed typically in a semi-formal language. There are two approaches to knowledge model specification, namely, starting with the inference knowledge and moving then to related domain and task knowledge, or starting with domain and task knowledge and linking these through inference rules. c) **Refinement**, in which validation of the knowledge model takes place.

The knowledge employed in PSIP can be considered as belonging in three categories:

d) **Domain knowledge**, in terms of types and facts, which is generally static. The domain schema is structured with concepts (i.e. classes), relations – associations, attributes (primitive values), and rule types (introducing expressions).
e) **Task knowledge**, in terms of functional decomposition, and control. In this regard, knowledge is elaborated with respect to combination of tasks to reach a

goal/workflow, or oppositely, decomposition of complex tasks into separate processes.

f) **Inference knowledge**, in terms of basic reasoning steps that can be made in the domain knowledge and are applied by tasks.

The proposed PSIP knowledge model architecture is depicted in Figure 1. The main component constitutes “ADE rules”. Its content is in the form of rules and is coupled with the content of the “Effects” component. The latter is the representation of all the effects which can result from a rule. The components “Drugs”, “Diagnosis”, “Lab results” and “Patient Parameters” are taxonomies which are used as terminology for expressing the rules. A first definition of “Context parameters” has been also elaborated.

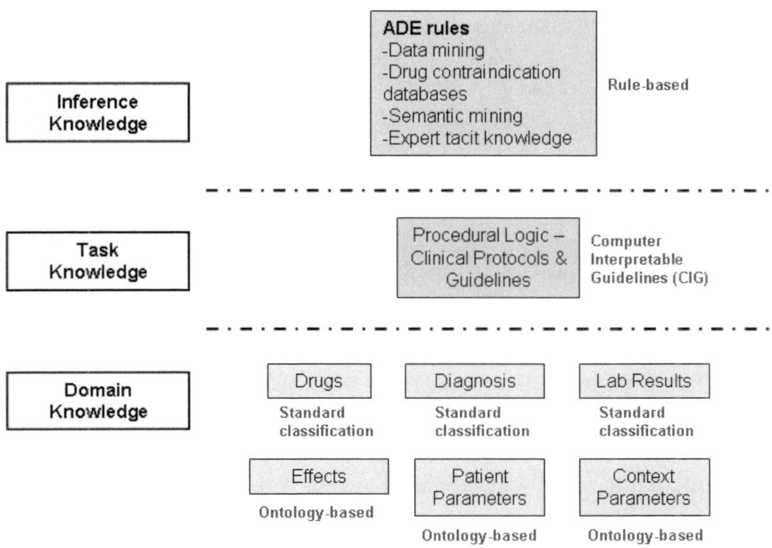

Figure 1. Knowledge model components in PSIP

More specifically, the components of the proposed Knowledge Model are the following:

a) *Drugs*: Definition of all possible drugs. It contains also categories and subcategories of drugs. The ATC (Anatomical Therapeutic Chemical) classification system is adopted for drug definition.

b) *Diagnosis*: Definitions of medical conditions, to be used as input parameters for identifying possible ADEs. The ICD-10 (International Classification of Diseases) standard classification is adopted for diagnosis definition.

c) *Lab results*: Defines the necessary terminology for expressing lab results in the “condition” part of ADE rules. The C-NPU (Committee on Nomenclature, Properties and Units) standard classification of IUPAC (International Union of Pure and Applied Chemistry) is adopted for lab results definition.

d) *Effects*: Ontology-based representation of the effects as entities. Several attributes are defined, which contain recommendation, level of severity, type of risk, etc. This component is actually a list of all possible effects that can be indicated as a result of an ADE.

e) *Patient parameters*: This component defines the necessary terminology for expressing the conditions of the ADE rules. It is a PSIP-specific ontology-based representation complying with the data model employed in the data mining procedure of the PSIP project.
f) *Context Parameters*: A set of context-related parameters defined to allow future contextualization for the CDSS modules.
g) *Procedural Logic – Clinical Protocols and Guidelines*: Description of clinical procedures, protocols and guidelines related to drugs. The main purpose is to be able to express knowledge related to human factors and complex ADE rules.
h) *ADE rules*: The core component containing knowledge about possible ADEs. The knowledge is in the form of rules associating a number of conditions to an effect (Figure 2). All previously described components are used as terminology for expressing ADE rules. Two levels of rules have been defined, main rules and intermediate rules.

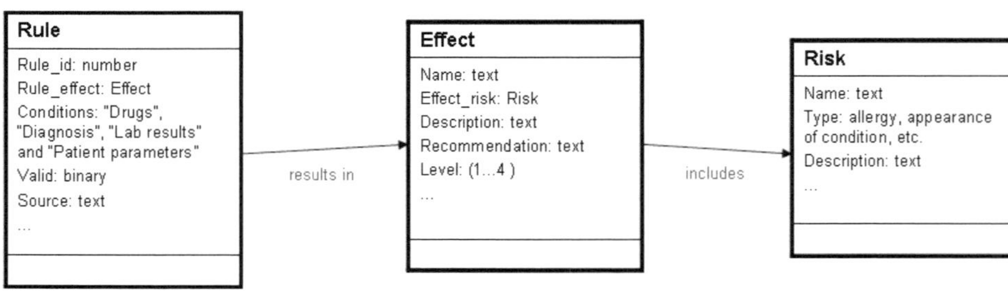

Figure 2. Class diagram of the "ADE rules" component

According to the above, the PSIP knowledge model is defined as a set of ontology-based structures, either PSIP-specific or standard classifications to be used as terminology. In addition, a rule-based component is included that is defined via a set of classes and populated with rules. The ontology-based structures and the rule-based component constitute the fundamental elements to define complex procedural logic in terms of protocols and guidelines, following an electronic formalism, i.e. the guideline modelling component. This formalism enables the unification of the former knowledge components into one single source, so as to provide a knowledge framework based on which the CDSS platform will offer its services.

6. Implementation Issues

The requirements and specifications for knowledge engineering presented, provided the foundations for the selection of the KBS for PSIP. An extensive investigation/evaluation phase followed, aiming to identify the appropriate candidate for PSIP, taking into account that the KBS will constitute the core of the CDSS platform for the project. The outcome of this task was the selection of GASTON, an IT technology tool developed for building tailor-made CDSSs. Its design is based on the so-called 'medical protocols', i.e. guidelines and working arrangements that describe how a physician or a nurse should act when treating patients. The core of the GASTON framework consists of a guideline representation formalism [15]. This formalism relies on a combination of knowledge representation approaches and concepts, i.e. primitives, problem-solving methods (PSMs) and ontologies. The representation uses ontologies as an underlying mechanism to represent guidelines in terms of PSMs and primitives in a consistent way. Two types of ontologies are defined, domain ontologies and method ontologies. Domain ontologies model domain-specific knowledge in terms of entities, attributes and relations, while method ontologies model concepts such as primitives, PSMs and guidelines similarly.

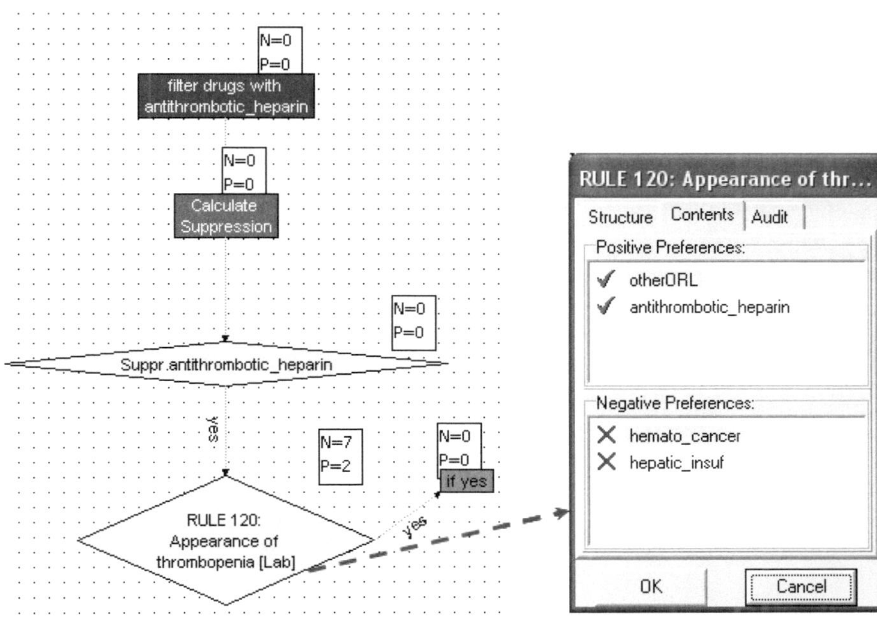

Figure 3. Example rule implementation

Up to now, initial experimentation with the system in a first development stage has been performed, so as to verify the applicability of the PSIP knowledge model in representing in practice the knowledge derived from the input sources. To this end, terminologies have been incorporated in the system and a number of representative example rules have been implemented. Figure 3 depicts the definition of the rule "*IF CDiag (cancer[hematology]) = 0 & CDiag (hepatic insufficiency) = 0 & DrugSuppr (heparin[antithrombotic]) = 0 & Drug (high weight heparin[antithrombotic]) = 1 & Drug (other ORL) = 1 THEN Appearance of Thrombopenia*" as guideline in GASTON. The rule combines diagnostic (denoted as *CDiag*) with drug variables (denoted as *Drug*) that, subject to appropriate "true" (indicated with *1*) or "false" (indicated with *0*) values, result in the appearance of thrombopenia. It has to be noted that rule conditions typically imply the construction of an intermediary rule, e.g. *Drug (other ORL) = 1* corresponds to a list of drugs indicated with ATC codes A12CX, R01AX10, R05X, etc.

7. Conclusion

The selection of the knowledge engineering approach and the design of the PSIP model have been primarily driven by the knowledge sources and the problem to be solved.

Although the value of developing a generic knowledge framework for ADE prevention is recognised, the domain is quite wide; thus, the path taken is starting from the knowledge currently available within the project and then appropriately extending the framework, so as to express additional sources of ADE knowledge. The result has been a knowledge framework tailored to the provided input, with a strong effort to maintain generality by defining its components in a generic way and by employing efficient and adequate knowledge representation formalisms and procedures. The next immediate step is to populate the model with knowledge, in order to construct an operational KB and evaluate the results. In this way, a feedback loop will be closed around the model construction process. Further challenges include the incorporation of more complex knowledge sources on ADEs, like knowledge related to human factors and tacit knowledge, as well as coping with contextualization of the KB.

Acknowledgment

The research leading to these results has received funding from the European Community's Seventh Framework Program (FP7/2007-2013) under Grant Agreement n° 216130 - the PSIP project (http://www.psip-project.eu/).

References

[1] D.W. Bates et al., Detecting adverse events using Information Technology, J Am Med Inform Assoc 10(2) (2003), 115–28.
[2] G. Schreiber, Knowledge Engineering, In: F. van Harmelen, V. Lifschitz, B. Porter (Eds.). Handbook of Knowledge Representation, Elsevier, 2008.
[3] H.J. Murff, V.L. Patel, G. Hripcsak and D.W. Bates, Detecting adverse events for patient safety research: A review of current methodologies, J Biomed Inform 36(1–2) (2003), 131–43.
[4] C. Bousquet, C. Henegar, A. Lillo-Le Louët, P. Degoulet and M.-C. Jaulent, Implementation of automated signal generation in pharmacovigilance using a knowledge-based approach, Int J Med Inform 74(7–8) (2005), 563–71.
[5] C. Henegar, C. Bousquet, A. Lillo-Le Louët, P. Degoulet and M.-C. Jaulent, Building an ontology of adverse drug reactions for automated signal generation in pharmacovigilance, Comput Biol Med 36(7–8) (2006), 748–67.
[6] I. Alecu, C. Bousquet, F. Mougin and M.C. Jaulent, Mapping of the WHO-ART terminology on SNOMED-CT to improve grouping of related adverse drug reactions, Stud Health Technol Inform 124 (2006), 833-8.
[7] V.L. Payne and D.P. Metzler, Hospital Care Watch (HCW): An ontology and rule-based intelligent patient management assistant, In: Proc. of the 18th IEEE CBMS Symp., 2005, pp. 479–84.
[8] S. Jeong and H.-G. Kim, Design of semantically interoperable adverse event reporting framework, In: The Semantic Web – ASWC 2006, Lecture Notes in Computer Science, vol. 4185, 2006, pp. 588-94, Springer-Verlag Berlin Heidelberg.
[9] M.A. Musen, Y. Shahar and E.H. Shortliffe, Clinical Decision-Support Systems, In: E.H. Shortliffe (Ed.). Biomedical Informatics: Computer Applications in Health Care and Biomedicine, 2006, Springer-Verlag, 2006.
[10] J.C. Wyatt, Management of explicit and tacit knowledge, J R Soc Med 94 (2001), 6–9.
[11] A. Gómez-Pérez, M. Fernández-López and O. Corcho, Ontological engineering, Springer-Verlag, 2004.

[12] A. Ligêza, Logical Foundations for Rule-Based Systems, Studies in Computational Intelligence, vol. 11, 2nd Ed., Springer-Verlag Berlin Heidelberg, 2006.
[13] P.A. de Clercq, J.A. Blom, H.H.M. Korsten and A. Hasman, Approaches for creating computer-interpretable guidelines that facilitate decision support, Artif Intell Med 31(1) (2004), 1–27.
[14] G. Schreiber et al., Knowledge Engineering and Management: The CommonKADS Methodology, MIT Press, 1999.
[15] P.A. de Clercq, A. Hasman, J.A. Blom and H.H.M. Korsten, Design and implementation of a framework to support the development of clinical guidelines, Int J Med Inform 64(2–3) (2001), 285–318.

Detection and Prevention of Adverse Drug Events
R. Beuscart et al. (Eds.)
IOS Press, 2009

doi:10.3233/978-1-60750-043-8-142

Strategy for Implementation and First Results of Advanced Clinical Decision Support in Hospital Pharmacy Practice

AMJW SCHEEPERS-HOEKS [a,1], RJE GROULS [a], C NEEF [b] and HHMKORSTEN [c]
[a] *Department of Pharmacy, Catharina-hospital Eindhoven, The Netherlands*
[b] *Department of Clinical Pharmacy and Toxicology, Maastricht University Medical Center, The Netherlands*
[c] *Department of Anesthesiology, Catharina-hospital Eindhoven, The Netherlands*

Abstract. Clinical decision support systems (CDSS) are the new generation clinical support tools that 'make it easy to do it right'. Despite promising results, these systems are not common practice, although experts agree that the necessary revolution in health care will depend on its implementation. To accelerate adoption a strategy is handed for structured development and validation of CDSS' content (clinical rules). The first results show that the proposed strategy is easily applicable for creating specific and reliable rules, generating relevant recommendations.

Keywords: Clinical decision support systems, clinical rules, medication safety, development, validation

Introduction

Medication errors occur disturbingly frequent due to deficiencies in the overall system of healthcare delivery, despite use of current medication safety systems [1-3]. Attention is called to the gaps between optimal and actual practice [1,2,4]. 'To err is human' made professionals and general public aware of the fact that 44.000 to 98.000 patients die in hospitals each year due to medical errors [2]. The following report 'Preventing Medication Errors' of the US Institute of Medicine (IOM) [4] showed that in the USA medications harm at least 1.5 million people each year of which at least 400,000 by preventable adverse drug events (ADE's) in hospitals. Therefore the IOM called seven years ago for a redesign of the healthcare delivery system [1]. One of the major goals, the nationwide implementation of an electronic medical record (EMR) by 2010, seems hard to reach as the process of adoption is slow. In fact, the use of an EMR marks only the beginning of a revolution in healthcare, because its availability is in fact only a prerequisite for the application of advanced clinical decision support systems (CDSS). These systems are the new generation clinical support tools for decision making that 'make it easy to do it right' [5]. CDSS are endorsed as one of the most powerful tools for improving patient safety and healthcare quality [1,2]. This is achieved by

[1] Corresponding Author: AMJW Scheepers-Hoeks, Catharina-hospital Eindhoven, Postbus 1350, 5602 ZA Eindhoven, The Netherlands; E-mail: anne-marie.scheepers@cze.nl

supporting clinical decision-making by matching patient characteristics to a computerized knowledge or rule base to generate patient-specific recommendations [6].

The urge for implementation of decision support is high, as in current practice medication errors are made frequently despite the use of drug-oriented medication safety systems [2,7]. These errors occur due to the rapidly increasing complexity of evidence based medicine and error sensitivity of healthcare [8]. Physicians need to take many drug- and patient specific characteristics into account and literature shows that this is often omitted or not recognized in time [3,9,10]. Another important cause of inefficiency is that current medication safety systems generate masses of irrelevant alerts causing clinicians to override most of the signals [11,12]. A CDSS can be a tool to overcome these problems. However, despite multiple opportunities and promising results, these systems are not yet common practice.

In our 600-bed university-affiliated hospital, we are on the eve of implementation of an advanced hospital-wide CDSS in practice (Gaston, Medecs, The Netherlands). The hospital has already implemented an Electronic Patient Record/Hospital Information System (EZIS, Chipsoft BV, Netherlands) including computerized physician order entry (CPOE) and medication safety alerting based on the Dutch drug standard (G-standaard, Royal Dutch Association for the Advancement of Pharmacy). An examination of the literature made clear which prerequisites are needed for optimal implementation of advanced CDSS. It was found that successful implementation of advanced CDSS depends on presenting information in the right message, at the right time, in the right place with the right system (table 1).

To accelerate the process of CDSS adoption, it is important to take the required success factors of CDSS into account. We found that the most important success factor is structured development and validation of CDSS' content (*clinical rules*). In this paper we will present our strategy for the development and validation leading to effective implementation of an advanced CDSS in hospital practice. Subsequently the first results collected by retrospective application of this strategy in pharmacy practice will be presented.

Table 1: Overview of success factors for implementation of CDSS

Right message	Accurate, reliable, understandable, actionable, including references
Right time	Integrated in workflow, time-saving, fast processing
Right place	Delivered at the point of care, right actor, active alerting
Right system	Electronic availability of data in the EMR, integrated with other systems, easy maintainable

1. Development and Validation Strategy for Clinical Rules

In our hospital, research is performed with clinical decision support since 1998, in which we developed a three-step strategy for development and validation of reliable clinical rules. In all three validation steps the Plan-Do-Check-Act cycle is followed, improving the quality of the clinical rule:

- PLAN: In this phase, the content of the clinical rule is developed or adjusted.
- DO: In the second phase the rule is tested on a database to generate the results

- CHECK: The results gathered in the previous phase are collected and interpreted to determine outcome values
- ACT: The results are discussed with an expert team, leading to the adjustments required for continuous improvement of the clinical rule. After this phase, the cycle is followed again until outcome values are optimised.

In every step the reliability and quality of the rule is expressed in a positive predictive value (PPV) and negative predictive value (NPV). The PPV is the amount of true positive alerts divided by the total amount of alerts. As true positives are the alerts that are technically correct and clinicallly relevant, the PPV is an indication of the reliability and usefulness of an alert. The NPV is the amount of true negatives divided by the total amount of patients without alerts and indicates if all patients that need a recommendation are seen by the CDSS.

1.1. Step 1: Technical Validation

The first step is a technical validation, to assure that the definitions in the clinical rule are correct and the parameters used in these definitions are linked to the correct data in the EMR.

First, the clinical rule is designed based on present evidence based guidelines or when unavailable other protocols or literature containing the best evidence on the subject. The challenge is to translate paper guidelines into a computer-interpretable format with measurable and specified parameters. Once the rule is developed, it is tested retrospectively on a large patient database containing at least one year of hospital data. Through review of the alerts generated by the clinical rule and comparing these with EMR-data, the alerts can be checked on technical correctness. The target value is a 100% technical correct link between CDSS and EMR to ensure that the clinical rule is exactly able to include and exclude the right patient and data (PPV). A NPV can be measured by using test cases or taking a random sample of patients without an alert. These cases can be taken to confirm that the rule is not applicable for these patients.

The calculated technical PPV and NPV are an indication of the technical correctness of the rule. Adjustment of possible flaws in mapping of parameters or definitions may be needed, aiming for a total technical accuracy of 100%.

1.2. Step 2: Therapeutic Validation

The second step is to verify that all alerts are clinically relevant, actionable and appreciated by end-users. This therapeutic validation is essential for gaining user acceptance. Although alerts generated are technically correct and based on evidence based guidelines, physicians may not want to receive the alert due to irrelevancy or non-actionable content. To overcome this, an expert team is required to fine-tune the clinical rule.

During therapeutic validation, the content of the clinical rule and the results of the first retrospective database test (step 1) are discussed with the expert team to determine the baseline therapeutic PPV and NPV. This enables to follow the progress of the predictive value during the development of the rule trough the development cycles. After this consultation, adjustments to the clinical rule are made, changes to the rule have to be technically validated first (step 1), before another PDCA-cycle is followed (step 2). In this cycle, every adjusted clinical rule is again tested and discussed with the expert team until the PPV and NPV are maximised.

The clinical rule at the end of this step is ready for retrospective use. When tested on a large database, these results can be used to measure the possible impact of the rule on medication safety. Hereby an impression can be given of what medication errors could have been prevented when the clinical rule had been active in the tested period. In the next paragraph some of our results after this step will be presented.

1.3. Step 3: Prospective Validation

The last step makes the clinical rule suitable for implementation in daily practice. In consultation with the expert team should be discussed what adjustments are necessary for presentation of the message in practice. Central point are: what should be the content of the message (e.g. proposal, command, automatic order), who will receive the message (e.g. nurse, physician, pharmacist), at what frequency/time (e.g. once daily, continuously) and with which specific alerting method should be used (e.g. on-demand, automatic).

Besides these additions, some rules require technical or content-related changes again before or after implementation in practice to optimise prospective use. For example, the rule has to be adjusted to react on certain triggers or a predefined frequency of testing during the day. These modifications have to be validated again through step 1 and 2, to guarantee technical and clinical validity.

In this step the rule is tested on a prospective database with patients admitted at the moment. We choose to generate a prospective Excel-list of all alerts, which can easily be validated daily to determine the final, prospective PPV and NPV. The clinical rule is now ready for bringing into practice.

2. Results

By application of the presented strategy, we developed dozens of clinical rules with a high predictive value [13-17]. All clinical rules developed so far have shown great progress in PPV and NPV values during the at least three PDCA-cycles. Baseline PPV's remained relatively low (average of 53%) due to the fact that the rule is not adapted to end-users wishes and technical disabilities. Eventually all final PPV's increased to a minimum of 94%, most rules having a PPV of 100%. This indicates that at least 94% of the messages generated are technically correct and clinical relevant. Also this shows that the multidisciplinary expert team has determined that at least 94% of the messages generated are desired by users of the system and that an action is indicated. Retrospective and prospective research has shown that with every clinical rule developed, a substantial increase in medication safety can be achieved.

An example is the clinical rule for lithium therapy [13]. In this complex rule patients using lithium are checked on laboratory values, drug dosing in elderly patients, interactions with other drugs, contra-indications etc. All these parameters derived from existing paper guidelines, but were not checked with our current medication safety system. Before application of the CDSS, the psychiatrist had to remember all the parameters that need to be checked according to the guidelines himself. After the first step, the PPV of the rule was 63%, rising to 83% after the first adjustments in step 2. Finally, after all technical and therapeutic adjustments, the PPV increased to 98%. This indicates that the strategy is able to increase the PPV during the cycles and optimise this value to a very high predictive value. Two years of retrospective database research has shown that the rule is also effective in detecting medication errors, defined as a correct alert given by the CDSS. We identified with this clinical rule 81 potentially adverse drug events (PADE's) in 71 patients in two years, that could have been prevented when the CDSS would have been active in that period.

Two more basic clinical rules are the rules for laxative use during opiods and gastric protection. The first had a baseline PPV of 56% that increased to 99% after three development cycles. Also the rule was easily applicable for detecting medication errors. Although it is easy to remember that when an opiod is prescribed, a laxative is indicated, this is founded to be omitted in 67% of the patients. The clinical rule for gastric protection enables addition of gastric protection in high risk patients using NSAIDs (see fig 1). This guideline in commonly known and can even partially be checked by the pharmacy with current basic systems. Nevertheless, in 40% of the patients a proton pump inhibitor is not prescribed, as detected by our CDSS through generation of alerts. The PPV of this rule rose to 100%, detecting all patients that need gastric protection in our hospital.

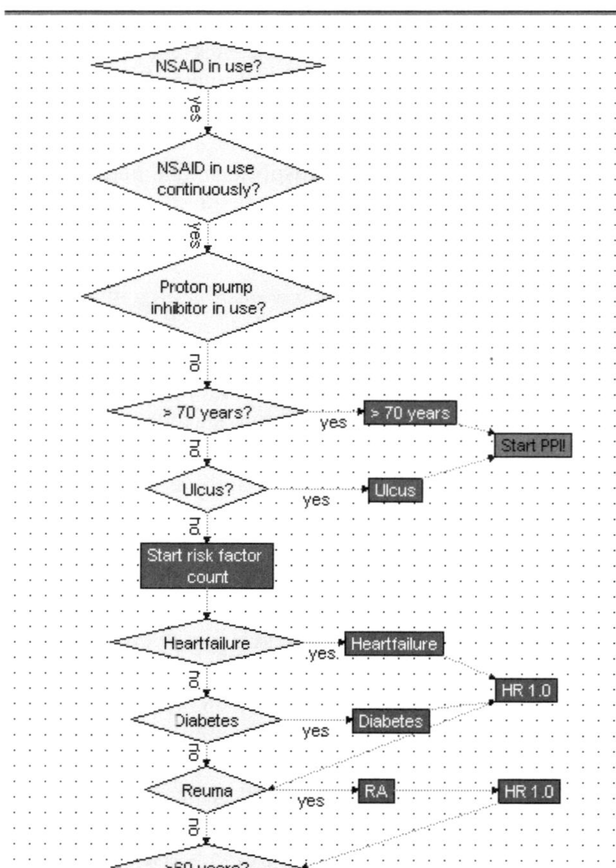

Figure 1: Part of the clinical rule for gastric protection, created in the CDSS Gaston (Medecs BV)

Another example is the clinical rule switch therapy, which detects patients that can be switched from intravenous to oral antibiotic therapy, as soon as the patient's condition improves [16]. Successful application of the strategy has led to an increase in PPV of 68% to 100%. Besides the increase in patient safety, this clinical rule can also reduce the length of hospitalization and lower associated costs. We found with retrospective research that in our hospital in one year, application of this rule can save approximately 17.000 euros. This financial benefit is due to earlier switching from intravenous to oral administrations, which have a significantly lower cost price. Other (financial) benefits are not taken into account in this estimation [16].

3. Discussion and Conclusion

In this paper a strategy is presented for the development and validation of clinical rules with a high predictive value. This strategy has led to the creation of new CDSS possibilities and refinement of definitions, which raised the predictive value of every clinical rule. The essential success factor of expert team consultation is included in the developed strategy. The first results show that this strategy is easily applicable for creating specific and reliable rules, generating relevant recommendations.

During the development of the strategy, the progression in PPV is followed with every clinical rule. Recently we added the measurement of NPV to strengthen the validation. This value is only determined explorative on a few clinical rules and therefore not included in the results. All negative validations have not shown false negative results so far, which leads to a NPV of 100%.

The strategy is applied on different clinical rules that are tested on at least one year of patient data, with approximately 15.000 patient records. The actual increase in medication safety of these clinical rules has yet to be confirmed in daily practice after prospective implementation.

This strategy has shown to be effective, as in all clinical rules the reliability expressed as PPV is equal or more than 94%. More research is needed to determine the minimum notification threshold for the predictive value of clinical rules and the variation in effect of different alert mechanisms. Together with this strategy, this will hopefully lead to standardisation and acceleration of the effective and widespread use of these promising next-generation decision support systems in daily practice.

References

[1] Committee on Quality of Health Care in America: Crossing the quality chasm: a new health system for the 21st century. Washington, D.C: National Academy Press; 2001

[2] Kohn L, Corrigan J, Donaldson M: To Err Is Human: Building a Safer Health System. Washington, DC: National Academy Press; 2000

[3] Schiff GD, Klass D, Peterson J, Shah G, Bates DW: Linking Laboratory and Pharmacy: Opportunities for Reducing Errors and Improving Care. Arch Intern Med 2003, 163: 893-900.

[4] Aspden P, Wolcott J, Bootman J, Cronenwett L: Preventing Medication Errors: Quality Chasm Series. Washington, DC: National Academy Press; 2006

[5] Garg AX, Adhikari NKJ, McDonald H, Rosas-Arellano MP, Devereaux PJ, Beyene J et al.: Effects of Computerized Clinical Decision Support Systems on Practitioner Performance and Patient Outcomes: A Systematic Review. JAMA 2005, 293: 1223-1238

[6] Kawamoto K, Houlihan CA, Balas EA, Lobach DF: Improving clinical practice using clinical decision support systems: a systematic review of trials to identify features critical to success. BMJ 2005, 330: 765

[7] Leendertse AJ, Egberts ACG, Stoker LJ, van den Bemt PMLA, for the HARM Study Group. Frequency of and Risk Factors for Preventable Medication-Related Hospital Admissions in the Netherlands. Arch Intern Med 2008; 168(17):1890-1896

[8] James B: Quality improvement opportunities in health care - Making it easy to do it right. J Manag Care Pharm 2002, 8: 394-399

[9] Denekamp Y: Clinical decision support systems for addressing information needs of physicians. Isr Med Assoc J 2007, 9: 771-776

[10] Levy M, Azaz-Livshits T, Sadan B, Shalit M, Geisslinger G, Brune K: Computerized surveillance of adverse drug reactions in hospital: implementation. Eur J Clin Pharmacol 1999, 54: 887-892.

[11] van der Sijs H, Aarts J, Vulto A, Berg M. Overriding of Drug Safety Alerts in Computerized Physician Order Entry. J Am Med Inform Assoc 2006; 13(2):138-147

[12] van der Sijs H, Aarts J, van Gelder T, Berg M, Vulto A. Turning Off Frequently Overridden Drug Alerts: Limited Opportunities for Doing It Safely. J Am Med Inform Assoc 2008; 15(4):439-448

[13] Wessels-Basten S, Hoeks A, Grouls R, Helmons P, Ackerman E, Korsten H: Development strategy and potential impact on medication safety for clinical rules: the lithium case. Br J Clin Pharmacol 2007, 63: 507-508.

[14] Helmons P, Grouls R, Roos A. The potential value on medication safety of a clinical decision support system in intensive care patients with renal insufficiency. Br J Clin Pharmacol 2007; 63(4):504.

[15] van Meijl FT, Paans JG, Scheepers-Hoeks AMJW, Mestrom M, Korsten HHM, Ackerman EW, Grouls RJE. Assessing the use of drugs contraindicated in hospitalized patients with heart failure using a CDSS: Development and validation of a clinical rule. Br J Clin Pharmacol 2009; 66(5):738.

[16] Paans JG, van Meijl FT, Scheepers-Hoeks AMJW, Mestrom M, Roos AN, Wulf MWH, Korsten HHM, Ackerman EW, Grouls RJE. Pharmacovigilance of intravenous-to-oral antibiotic switch therapy: Development and validation of a clinical rule. Br J Clin Pharmacol 2009; 66(5):740.

[17] Paans JG, van Meijl FT, Scheepers-Hoeks AMJW, Mestrom M, Korsten HHM, Grouls RJE. Pregnancy, an unrecognised contraindication: Development and validation of a clinical rule. Br J Clin Pharmacol 2009; 66(5):740.

Detection and Prevention of Adverse Drug Events
R. Beuscart et al. (Eds.)
IOS Press, 2009

doi:10.3233/978-1-60750-043-8-149

Inevitable Components of and Steps for ADE Management Systems: The Need for a Unified Ontological Framework (UOF)[1] and a More Effective Collaboration in Medication Safety

Esat N. ERYILMAZ [a, 2], Gül DÜNDAR [3] and Senem Özgür SARI [b]
[a] *Retired from University*
[b] *Anadolu Health Center, Pharmacy Director*

Abstract. In this article, we will try to address the most basic requirements for facilitating the knowledge management challenges through the elaboration of medical documentation/ record keeping with several implications on patient safety/medication safety and research quality aspects, the main purpose being the simplification of utilizing the usable outputs of ontology development efforts. This simplification is of vital importance from KM implementation in medical and healthcare domains. Because, as Ceusters et al [3] elaborate, reaching consensus on even the most basic concepts will become an intricate work in terms of the wide-scale implementation of ontology-based KM solutions in clinical practice and other healthcare related processes. EHR (Electronic Health Records) standards developed by various SDOs[4] are not easy to implement in all circumstances. Any implementation effort, not complying with a UOF (Unified Ontological Framework), is likely to fail in terms of goal-oriented optimization and high quality safe medical practice. World- wide trend is to standardize medical documents focusing on the use of terminology systems covering care related processes.

Keywords. Ontology Implementation, unified ontological framework, patient safety and HCICT, knowledge management in healthcare, Adverse Drug Events, Drug-induced medical errors, clinical outcomes management, medical ontology requirements specifications

Introduction

"Health" and "Being Healthy" or Maintaining Health" is a very complex and dynamic issue. Designing appropriate healthcare environment, providing health services and clinical practice are also very complex aspects of health systems, the reason being the inter-disciplinary and inter-professional nature of health service at the point-of-care.

---

1 UOF: Unified Ontological Framework (The definition by the Authors)
2 Corresponding Author: Esat Nadir ERYILMAZ, Healthcare Process Engineering Consultant esatnadir@gmail.com, esat_eryilmaz@yahoo.co.uk
3 Reyhan Eczanesi, Bostanci-Istanbul
4 SDOs: Standards Development Organizations

The most critical and complex aspect of health system is the "Knowledge Management" throughout the healthcare chain. This inherent complexity is being addressed in various scientific meetings [5] and Special Issues of domain publications[6].

On the other hand, "Healthcare" is claimed to be the largest industry in the world [1]. As Vincent [1] puts: '...Healthcare is even larger then military in spending, numbers of people employed, use of use of resources and the wider impact on the population at large. It is, in addition, extraordinarily diverse in terms of the activities involved and the way it is delivered.' Healthcare is characterized by rising costs and climbing expectations as to the quality and safety of services provided in addition to critical issue of timeliness.

The interest shown by diverse disciplines and health professionals, in addition to great numbers of professionals from other disciplines/domains (computer scientists, cognitive scientists, economists politicians, various engineering disciplines, management professionals, lawyers, linguists etc...) towards medical errors and unintended consequences which are considered to be healthcare-associated has increased significantly compared to the professional efforts aiming to put scientific, technical and medical evidence in practice. Efforts and resources assigned to patient safety issues primarily focus on implementing and deploying process-oriented approaches together with workflow management (WFM) capabilities in healthcare provider organizations. From the point of WFM functionalities, compliance to clinical guidelines (CGL) and care maps at the point-of-care still needs to be addressed through medico-legal and ethical perspectives including patient rights as to privacy and confidentiality.

The implicit underlying causes of this trend are, but not limited to, as follows: (1) Ongoing problems in consolidating patient and healthcare-related data/information, major reasons being the lack of a "unified ontological framework (UOF)" and un-regulated terminology system [7] (results, findings, clinical outcomes, clinical performance indicators, prognoses, ADEs, complications etc...); (2) At world-wide scale, problems in sharing "clinical evidence" and "unintended consequences", which are of complete psycho-social nature; (3) Unavailability of integrated information systems applications with satisfying functionalities at affordable costs; (4) Clinical performance management issues are not treated properly based on scientifically proven tools, with the exception of recent meetings and publications [8].

Better healthcare with better outcomes has been on top of communities' priorities in their health systems' agendas in addition to promoting healthcare and preventing

---

5 Second Call for invited Papers, Methodology of Societal Complexity, The 23rd European Conference on Operational Research, EURO XXIII, Bonn, 2009, Germany , Europe July 5- 8 2009; http://www.euro-2009.de/ Main Stream 10 Health, life sciences & bioinformatics on Methodology of Societal Complexity consists of: Session I: Societal Complexity and Safety; Session II: Societal Complexity and Sustainable Development; Session III: Societal Complexity and Healthcare

6 Announcement: Journal of Biomedical Informatics 41 (2008) 861–862 Call for Papers: Biomedical Complexity and Error Special Issue; Guest Editors: Vimla L. Patel, Ph.D., D.Sc., Director, Center for Decision Making and Cognition, Department of Biomedical Informatics, Arizona State University; Kanav Kahol, Ph.D., Manager, Human Machine Symbiosis Laboratory, Assistant Professor, Department of Biomedical Informatics, Arizona State University; Timothy Buchman, M.D., Ph.D., Edison Professor of Surgery Professor of Anesthesiology and of Medicine, Washington University School of Medicine; Submission Deadline: February 1, 2009

7 Founding efforts of IAOA (International Appied Ontology Association) are under way. http://www.loa-cnr.it/Location.html).

8 Health Care Benchmarking and Performance Evaluation An Assessment using Data Envelopment Analysis (DEA) Yaşar A. ÖZCAN Springer, 2008

diseases. Ageing population, late diagnoses, drug utilization issues, drug-induced "Adverse Events" and failures in assuring availability of relevant information at the point of care in clinical contexts increases the burden of disease throughout the world.

At all stages and in every step of providing care, good planning and provision constitutes the backbone of quality healthcare. The inevitable constituents of quality healthcare and patient safety are: (1) Expert teams of inter-professional working culture, (2) Patient data (current and longitudinal) complying Semantic Interoperability Requirements, (3) Scientific evidence (Relevant information from the scientific corpora), (4) Risk assessment and management capabilities of care teams, (5) Knowledge sharing behavior of care-team members and patient data providers (institutions), (6) Ethical profiles of team members and codes of ethics, (7) Physical conditions at the point of care enabling clean care.

Ethical and medico-legal frameworks are determined by government regulations together with professional and ethical principles. While technologies of all kinds and complexities (inc. internet) have been around us for years, knowledge and information acquisition, compliant with semantic interoperability requirements, has stayed immature despite multi-national, multi-disciplinary and inter-professional efforts.

Buzzoni [2] claims that "...the new awareness has grown that a full comprehension of medical praxis is impossible without integrating its scientific status with phenomenological and hermeneutic aspects". Among the constituents of care quality and patient safety scientific evidence and patient data play a crucial role, and one should consider the barriers against this availability. Availability of relevant and accurate data is very important while the same availability may cause to grave results and outcomes due to irrelevant and inaccurate data/information.

Beyond shared EPRs, EHRs, EMRs and even PHRs a common repository of medication side effects (known and documented), unexpected complications (due to drug use) and other adverse events through care praxis must be shared among the care providers according to patient consent, legal/ethical frameworks and finally regional/national and international patients' rights declarations.

Data and information ownership issues, in this context of crucial importance, form the most important barrier in assuring care quality and patient safety in addition to enterprise vocabulary/ontology [9] services. Other critical barrier has been the common behavior of overlooking Clinical Guidelines and Care Pathways. Establishing a virtual standard ontology services for healthcare (covering all nomenclatures and taxonomies of practical value in medical praxis, mappings etc...) is considered to be the most fundamental common action for an international semantic interoperability framework.

In this article, we will try to address the most basic requirements for facilitating the knowledge management challenges through the elaboration of medical documentation/ record keeping with several implications on patient safety/medication safety and research quality aspects, the main purpose being the simplification of utilizing the usable outputs of ontology development efforts. This simplification is of vital importance from KM implementation in medical and healthcare domains. Because, as Ceusters et al [3] elaborate, reaching consensus on even the most basic concepts will become an intricate work in terms of the wide-scale implementation of ontology-based KM solutions in clinical practice and other healthcare related processes.

---

[9] Supporting e-trials over distributed networks: a tool for capturing randomized controlled trials (RCT) eligibility criteria using the National Cancer Institute´s (NCI) Enterprise Vocabulary Services (EVS) ARVANITIS T, 12th Mednet 2007 World Conference in Leipzig, Germany

1. Information Infrastructure Framework at the Point-of-Care

In order to emphasize the main point of this writing, confusing jargon developed so far (EMR, EPR, CPR, CMR, PHR, CIS, HIS, POMR, Medical IS [10]) shall not be elaborated in detail. The definition and conceptual framework of "Hospital Information Systems" should be re-evaluated and this intricate task should be effected through the adoption Medical Information Systems and Healthcare Resource Planning (HRP) instead of Enterprise Resource Planning (ERP), with semantic interoperability standards (if any and if applicable) and UOF-Compliant (UOF: Unified Ontological Framework) outcome classification/reporting systems. This approach requires a different approach for the organization and management of healthcare practice, with special emphasis on CoC (Continuity of Care) according to patient-centered, process-based perspectives. Primary processes a healthcare organization expected to perform are diagnosis of diseases and treatment accordingly.

Point of Care could be any point, location and context throughout the health system. Therefore, semantic interoperability is very important in many respects: (1) Timely and accurate diagnosis of disease, (2) Treatment effectiveness, (3) Achieving the world-wide goal of better and safer care with less resource, (4) Increasing research quality, (5) Reducing medical errors resulting better patient safety achievements.

Delivering health care services does not take place within the product-tree framework. All healthcare services, related processes and sub-processes including interventions are contextual. GST (General Systems Theory) and WST (Work Systems Theory) should be applied to healthcare provider organizations. But the most important undertaking before GST and WST's application and deployment to health systems, is making a UOF (Unified Ontological Framework) operational and obligatory. This attitude will pave the way for semantic interoperability, if all the steps taken properly.

1.1. Conceptual Framework Towards a Consistent Outcome Classifications: Applicability and Simplicity

EHR (Electronic Health Records) standards developed by various SDOs[11] are not easy to implement in all circumstances. Any implementation effort, not complying with a UOF, is likely to fail in terms of goal-oriented optimization and high quality safe medical practice. World- wide trend is to standardize medical documents focusing on the use of terminology systems covering care related processes[12]. Mandatory utilization and compliance to UOF must/shall cover:

- ERS (Error Reporting System) awareness training to all health professionals (Attitudes of healthcare professionals to error reporting, case studies for worldwide reporting systems implementation, examples of error classification systems

---

[10] **EMR**: Electronic Medical Records, **EPR**: Electronic Patient Records, **CPR**: Computerized Medical Records, **CPR**: Computerized Patient Records, **PHR**: Personal Health Records, **CIS**: Clinical Information Systems, **HIS**: Hospital Information Systems, **POMR**: Problem Oriented Medical records, **Medical IS**: Medical Information Systems

[11] SDOs: Standards Development Organizations

[12] Health Info-way Project of Canada, e-MS Implementation Component (e-MS: Electronic Medical Summary), Arztbrief in Germany

- Stratification of conceptual dimensions in UOF for pragmatic benefits and adoption of standard outcome classifications inc. ADE and XCU complications (XCU: various ICU environments such as Paediatric, neonatal, surgical, coronary etc)
- Error Reporting System implementation training: Requirements, Design, Verification, Validation, Usability, Operational and Maintenance aspects
- Well-structured quality and safety training with special emphasis on the observability of clinical outcomes and partial/holistic performance
- Patient Risk Management and Clinical Decision Support Functionalities training
- Cross-mapping of existing nomenclatures, classifications and coding systems to UOF (Medical practice, care monitoring, re-imbursement, cost optimization, GL-compliance aspects, CoC applicability and minimum conditions, ...)
- Developing WFM and BPM capabilities in healthcare institutions within diverse clinical clinical specialties

Since its inception of health informatics, approximately 40 years have elapsed and the contributions of associated fields of practice are not considered to be of expected level in terms of health outcomes obtained through clinical practice, except the unexpected numbers and varieties of medical errors. In [4], Pisanelli and Gangemi looks at the current status of promises and pitfalls of ontologies, including related tools and methodologies, within a more general health informatics context. Ceusters et al [5] questions the origins of mistakes in medical ontologies, which emphasise the critical importance and fundamental requirement as to an UOF (Unified Ontological Framework). UOF, by definition, is a dynamic, pragmatic, flexible clusters of concepts in a clinical context (PoC), its linguistic elements being in complete compliance with all domain ontologies under consideration for the specific clinical context at the specified PoC. Among the domains under consideration are drug utilization codes (ATC, vetATC), procedure coding systems, GS1 Healthcare classification systems, accepted problem lists in various medical specialty areas etc.

According to the authors of this article the most fundamental requirement for an adoptable and deployable KM application in clinical practice and medicine is a dynamic, comprehensive and consistent concept clusters (UOF) enabling to keep record of the outcomes of every category in their interests. The vital importance of an adoptable and deployable KM application is dictated by rising costs of healthcare and reluctance in evidence-based clinical practice, indeed. Medical disciplines and specialties including other healthcare professions urgently require a common comprehension interface as to the outcomes such as complications of various origins and proven deterministic relations between diagnostic and therapeutic procedures in well-defined definite clinical contexts. However, they are known not to show, to a considerable extent, an interest to domain specific meta-level discourse areas. (Knowledge engineering, knowledge acquisition, knowledge representation etc...) Issues like human and organizational dynamics in e-Health, socio-technical aspects of medical information systems development, clinical systems implementation do not even seem to have significant impacts on clinical practice and information seeking behaviors of most health professionals.

Although the primary concern of this article is not to address the KM-induced implementation problems, one should admit that all implementation failures and challenges are influenced by the lack of an error-free ontological framework, namely "Unified Ontological Framework". Another study on Ontological Representation Framework concept is being conducted by the first author of this article to position the acceptability and deployment capabilities of UOF in the medical domain[13]. The lack of such an understanding, especially among medical professional professions, hinders the adoptability and deployment of ontology-based KM applications in healthcare. Wennerberg et al [6] distinguishes between two different types of knowledge engineering challenges, the first one being the communication process between the knowledge engineer and the medical expert and the second being specifically about the engineering of medical ontologies. According to the authors of this article, the real problem is the lack of an acceptable/applicable terminological interface between the ontologies used and methodologies utilized, in addition to the contextual information set(s) subject to evaluation at the point of care and in a clinical context.

To further elaborate the UOF concept, consider the following discussion: Among the various medical and healthcare related domain ontologies intra- and inter- domain linking and editing methodologies/tools, there exist only two prime types of information clusters from patient safety and clinical efficiency/effectiveness perspectives. The members/elements of these clusters cannot simply be treated as one dimensional propositions/statements associated with contextual clinical conditions (patient status), previously proven deterministic relations for a specific patient. Wennerberg et al continues by mentioning two prominent problems: (1) KE[14]-specific challenges and (2) KA[15]-bottleneck [6]. In our opinion, these KE-specific challenges and KA-bottleneck stipulated by Wennerberg et al [6] are mainly caused by the lack of mature methodological processes at "Dynamic Outcomes" cluster within OUF. In order to assure a seamless interoperability and inter-professional, inter-disciplinary comprehension in this cluster of concept, a UOF is a must for significant scientific advancements and progress in other related fields (HCICT, pharmaceutical industry, regulatory bodies, SDOs[16], medical technology suppliers such as PYXIS in the medication management area, healthcare providers, academia, …).

Let us consider the KM-Framework for relevant functionalities at PoC, given the access rights made operational within legal and ethical concerns (Figure 1.).

[13] A survey on critical data and information sharing issues in clinical practice is being conducted, with a target number of **1000** healthcare professionals, in parallel to ORF study (ORF: Ontological Representation Framework in Medical Domain).

[14] KE: Knowledge Engineering

[15] KM: Knowledge Management

[16] SDO: Standards Development Organizations

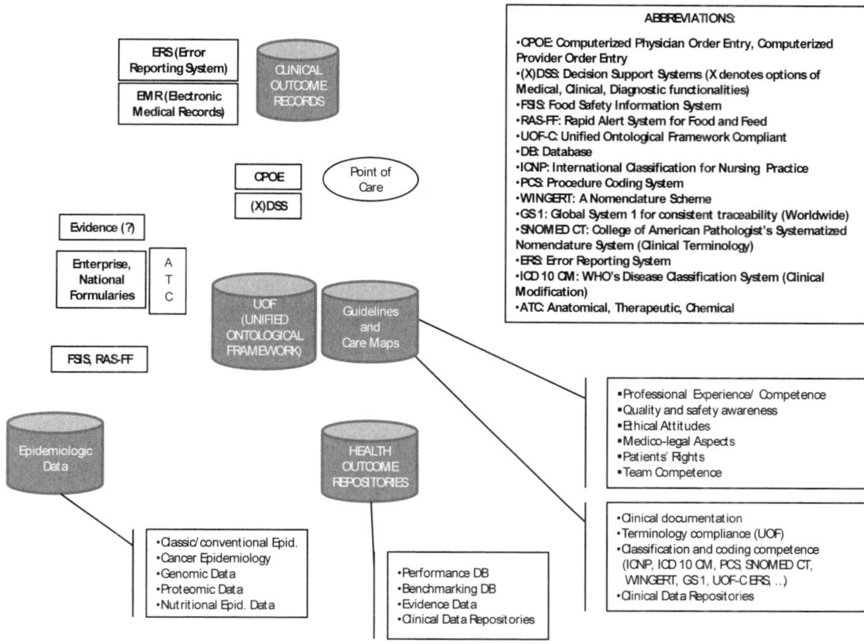

Figure 1. Information Infrastructure at the Point-of-Care.

We are to consider the following critical questions in the context of PoC (Point of Care) and systems' and information/data services availability:

- How many systems are to be utilized for better and safer care?
- Is it practical and/or applicable to exhaust the capabilities of the individual databases and systems for better and safer care?
- Are the support systems and information resources adopted by healthcare team's members in the context of patient care?
- Do Healthcare team's members cover medical record competencies and relevant experience?

1.2. Point of Care Information Needs, Attitudes to Information Use, and Maturity of Information Systems

Technology, with capabilities and features beyond organizational and professional expectations, has always been around us, unfortunately with less contributions to and improvements in the ways healthcare services organized and provided. One of the reasons for this case has been the inherent irrelevance of information services infrastructure(s). This irrelevance can be explained in two respects: One is the complex nature of the healthcare itself, the other being the omitting of this complexity at the requirements elicitation phase of system(s) development. But the hidden cause of information systems failures in healthcare domain is the lack of a unified ontological framework covering all aspects of medicine and healthcare related domains, including health problems RFE, RFH, RFR, RFM [17] and outcomes. RFEs, RFHs, RFRs, RFMs and other information sets are produced at the junction points of HCC (Healthcare Chain) throughout the entire health system. These junctions are the most relevant starting points of semantic interoperability. A detailed account of the failures and insufficiencies of semantic interoperability is out of the scope of this writing. It should be given a high priority among the next activities intending to enable an effective collaboration in the field of patient safety with special on medication safety and medication errors.

In this paragraph, we elaborate, to some extent only, the impact of not using a UOF as a common professional communication and comprehension.

Acceptance of a common communication framework, at least at sub-categorical levels, should be deemed essential as a prerequisite for semantic interoperability; and compliance to this ontological framework should be regulated and audited very strictly, to enable consolidation of collected data/information throughout clinical practice and health system's entirety. For example, DDI [18] and DFI [19] are considered and/or understood to be anatomical, physiological, patho-anatomical and patho-physiological" processes taking place in human body depending upon the patient's status and health-care related interventions (diagnostic, therapeutic, care-related, monitoring associated) in clinical contexts. Multiple combinations of DDI, DFI and DL_DI[20], L_DFI[21] are no exceptions to tihis evaluation. (L_D: Latent-drugs contained in foodstuff). Outcomes of those interactions, individually or in combination with each other, conform the most relevant scientific and medical evidence if recorded according to a UOF for consolidation and conclusions.

1.3. An Approach to Unification and Simplification of Clinical Classifications and Health Information Records

Semantic categorization of "ADE" concept itself is another issue of critical importance within semantic interoperability and evidence based practice contexts. ADEs are outcomes associated with inter-related clinical processes and interventions, some of them being influenced by re-imbursement rules and health insurance schemes. Parallel to this, complications encountered in ICU (Intensive Care Unit) are all outcomes resulting from:

- Patient's current status & conditions
- Decisions made and applied by healthcare professionals
- Data/Information Quality, available during clinical interventions (Lab results, ATC/DDD[22] indications, UOF compliance, etc…)

An ADE (Adverse Drug Events) cannot and should not be considered as a "PROCESS" in healthcare contexts. Because it is the resultant outcome encountered in a patient, in a definite clinical context evolved through a set of HC environmental conditions and interventional processes/sub-processes. The dimensions of medical errors within a

---

[17] **RFE**: Reason for Encounter, **RFH**: Reason for Hospitalization, **RFR**: Reason for Referral, **RFM**: Reason for Medication

[18] **DDI**: Drug-drug Interaction

[19] **DFI**: Drug-Food Interaction

[20] **DL_DI**: Drug-Latent Drug Interaction (**L_D** = Latent Drug in Foodstuff)

[21] **L_DFI**: Latent Drug-Food Interaction (**L_D** = Latent Drug in Foodstuff)

[22] **ATC**: Anatomical Therapeutic Chemical **DDD**: Defined Daily Dose

UOF are different from ADEs. A multi-dimensional, trans-disciplinary, inter-professional viewpoint is necessary, even compulsory, for a scientifically, linguistically relevant positioning of medical errors and ADEs, with achievements to a high degree of semantic interoperability and medical advancement. This multi-dimensionality must comply with a Unified Healthcare Ontology Framework, which is proposed as a starting point for a world-wide semantic interoperability.

2. A Roadmap for UOF-Compliant Clinical Outcomes Repository

As the scientific basis for evidence-based medical practice, designing and developing a UOF-compliant clinical outcomes repository is the most immediate step. PSIP project and its components are indications of this requirement. UOF-compliance should be an integral part of each and every PSIP project component. Ensuring this integrity necessitates the work packages listed in Table 1.

Table 1. Work Packages for Ensuring The UOF-Compliance in Medication Safety-Oriented System Development Projects

Work Package Description	Possible Stekeholders	Suggested Priority Among Project Work Packages
[1] Privacy and confidentiality requirements framework development	All Project Participants	Very High
[2] Distinction and clarification of process ownership and data ownership according to GST and WST approaches in compliance with [1]	All Project Participants and Stakeholders in Health System	High
[3] Developing a security policy document based on privacy and confidentiality requirements (See Work Package [1])	All Project Participants and Stakeholders in Health System	Very High
[4] Developing a UOF for implementation in selected clinical settings and disease groups (Critical Care and Peri-operative environment)	All Project Participants and Stakeholders in Health System	Very Very High/MUST
[5] Identification, clarification, validation and verification of ADE monitoring/Reporting requirements in selected/prioritized clinical settings	All Project Participants and Stakeholders in Health System	Very Very High/MUST
[6] Methodology training for ensuring UOF-compliance in selected implementation projects	All Project Participants and Stakeholders in Health System	High
[7] Designing and developing a semantically interoperable system for a UOF-compliant clinical outcome repository	All Project Participants and Stakeholders in Health System	Very Very High/MUST

3. Conclusion

"The recent growth in the scientific understanding of diseases and their management has been unprecedented, but has not been matched by an equivalent ability to apply that knowledge in practice. It is now humanly impossible for unaided healthcare professionals to deliver patient care with the efficacy, consistency and safety that the full range of current knowledge could support" [7]. Failures in integrating and consolidating medical information require a common regulated but dynamic/flexible ontological framework for diffusion of innovations [8]. However, necessary competence in KM and information utilization has not reached to an acceptable and deployable maturity, one of the major reasons being the lack of a common comprehension framework in relation to developed ontologies and related tools and methodologies. An implementation framework is treated in this article, with special emphasis on medication safety, and a UOF (Unified Ontological Framework) is proposed to facilitate the implementation of interoperable medical information systems throughout the health systems. Clarification of formal requirements as to the specifications of UOF in clinical practice and healthcare supply chain is the next major task for verification and validation; tasks of priority, with assigned estimations are mentioned in the article, to a limited extent.

Solving the medical knowledge crisis in the context of Open Clinical's whitepaper and today's public health urgencies require the KM way of professional practice in many respects [10].

References

[1] C. VINCENT, Patient Safety, Elsevier-Churchill Livingstone, Toronto, 2006.

[2] M. BUZZONI, On Medicine as a Human Science, Theoretical Medicine and Bioethics Vol 24(1), 2003 pp.79

[3] W. CEUSTERS, M. CAPOLUPO, G. DE MOOR, Jos DEVLIES, Introducing Realist Ontology for the Representation of Adverse Events. 237-250. In: Formal Ontology in Information Systems, C. Eschenbach and M. Grüninger (Eds.) Proc. Of the Fifth International Conference (FOIS 2008) IOS Press, Amsterdam, 2008.

[4] Domenico M. PISANELLI, Aldo GANGEMI, If Ontology is the Solution, What is the Problem? In: Ontologies in Medicine, IOS Press, Amsterdam Ed. Domenico M Pisanelli 2004, 1-19.

[5] Werner CEUSTERS, Barry SMITH, Anand KUMAR, Christoffel DHAEN Mistakes in Medical Ontologies: Where do they come from and How Can They Be Detected? In: Ontologies in Medicine, IOS Press, Amsterdam Ed. Domenico M Pisanelli 2004, 145-163.

[6] Pinar WENNERBERG, Sonja ZILLNER, Manual MÖLLER, Paul BUITELAAR, Michael SINTEK, KEMM: A Knowledge Engineering Methodology in the Medical Domain, 79-91. In: Formal Ontology in Information Systems, C. Eschenbach and M. Grüninger (Eds.) Proc. Of the Fifth International Conference (FOIS 2008) IOS Press, Amsterdam, 2008.

[7] Open Clinical White Paper: The medical knowledge crisis and its solution through knowledge management at http://www.openclinical.org/ Accessed on April 23rd, 2009.

[8] J. David JOHNSON, Innovation and Knowledge Management – The Cancer Information Service Research Consortium , Edward Elgar, Chelthenham, UK 2005.

[9] Michael E. HOBART and Zachary S. SCHIFFMAN, Information Ages – Literacy, Numeracy, and the Computer Revolution, The Johns Hopkins University Press, Baltimore 1998.

[10] Hubert SAINT-ONGE, Debra WALLACE, Leveraging Communities of Practice for Strategic Advantage, Butterworth-Heinemann, Amsterdam 2003.

Detection and Prevention of Adverse Drug Events
R. Beuscart et al. (Eds.)
IOS Press, 2009

doi:10.3233/978-1-60750-043-8-159

Computerised Physician Order Entry (CPOE)

Anne Regitze HARTMANN HAMILTON [a, 1], Jacob ANHØJ [a], Annemarie HELLEBEK [a], Jonas EGEBART [a], Brian BJØRN [a] and Beth LILJA [a]
[a] *The Unit for Patient Safety, Capital Region of Denmark, Kettegård Alle 30, Dept. 023, 2650 Hvidovre, Denmark*

Abstract. The purpose of this study is to examine how everyday use of the Computerised Physician Order Entry (CPOE) system in the Capital Region of Denmark has led to medication errors. The study is based on clinicians' reporting of patient safety incidents. It was found that the immediate causes of the patient safety incidents primarily relates to a) a mismatch between clinical work routines and the structure of the CPOE system, b) the complexity of the user interface, and c) lack of barriers against commonly occurring, severe errors in some areas of the CPOE system. The following was concluded: A well designed CPOE system should be intuitive, provide barriers against serious mistakes, and make the correct choice an easy one. Furthermore it was concluded that it is important that the CPOE system closely supports accepted clinical work routines and that risk assessment is performed prior to implementing new design or functionality.

Keywords. Patient safety, Computerised Physician Order Entry, patient safety incident, medication error, documentation.

Introduction

The implementation of the Computerised Physician Order Entry (CPOE) system in the Capital Region of Denmark is an ongoing process that began in 2005.

The CPOE system – which covers only the medication process – includes functionality for prescribing and dispensing drugs as well as bar code scanners for use in the administration process.

The transition from documenting patients' medication on paper forms to the use of CPOE has eliminated certain types of errors such as illegible hand writing and transcription errors. However, reports of patient safety incidents relating to the use of CPOE suggest that the complexity of the system has led to the occurrence of other types of errors. The purpose of this study is therefore to examine how the everyday use of CPOE has led to medication errors as well as near-misses.

1. Material

This study is based on reports of patient safety incidents relating to the everyday use of CPOE. Reports derived from larger system outages are therefore not included.

[1] Corresponding Author.

The reports were identified from a database search on the term "EPM" (Danish translation of the acronym "CPOE") for the period 1 January, 2007 till 30 September, 2008, representing all hospitals in the Capital Region of Denmark. Reports were excluded where the term was coincidently mentioned but the incident otherwise had no relation to the CPOE system. Both actual medication errors and near-misses were included due to an equal learning potential. As a means of limiting the quantity of results retrieved, only patient safety incidents pre-categorised as actual or potentially serious were included. Altogether 300 reports of incidents were included in this study.

The reports were submitted by clinicians in a non-controlled fashion and may therefore be subject to reporting bias. The number of submitted reports covers only an (unknown) portion of the actual number of patient safety incidents. Due to these constraints, the focus of this study is placed on the issues raised by the reports, rather than the actual number of reports.

2. Methods

The reports of patient safety incidents were pre-classified by each hospital according to actual and potential patient harm resulting from the incident. For the purpose of this study, reports were further categorised according to:

- Where in the medication process the patient safety incident took place
- The type of medication error
- The immediate cause of the patient safety incident (as opposed to the root cause, which is unknown unless a root cause analysis was performed).

The clinicians' assessment as to the cause of a patient safety incident has not been further interpreted in this report. As such there could be differing opinions between the system users and CPOE experts as to the immediate cause of an incident.

3. Results

Regarding patient harm, none of the 300 patient safety incidents were pre-categorised as having caused disastrous patient harm. 5% caused significant patient harm, 32% moderate patient harm, and 63% minimal or no patient harm at all. The less serious incidents were included in the study because they potentially could have caused serious patient harm (but for various reasons did not).

46% of the patient safety incidents occurred in relation to the prescription process, 24% in relation to the dispensing process, 3 % in relation to administering the medicine, 23% relating to documentation, and 4% without the possibility of determining in which part of the medication process the incident took place.

This study focuses mainly on the causes of incidents since issues identified through this approach could be useful in future efforts to improve the CPOE system.

The immediate causes of the patient safety incidents represent three main issues:

- A mismatch between clinical work routines and the structure of the CPOE system

- The complexity of the user interface of the CPOE system
- Lack of barriers against commonly occurring, severe errors in some areas of the CPOE system

3.1. Clinical Work Routines and the Structure of the CPOE System

This includes cases of parallel documentation (CPOE and paper forms; CPOE and other electronic medication systems) that typically resulted in doses being administered twice or missed doses.

Lack of flexibility in the CPOE system regarding prescriptions that require flexible dosing (according to a lab value) or flexible time of administration (according to the time of surgery) are other examples of a mismatch between the structure of the CPOE system and clinical work routines.

When a patient is transferred from one hospital ward to another, re-approval of his or her prescribed medication is required by a doctor in the new ward before it can be administered to the patient. Logistical problems in relation to this procedure were seen to cause delays in the medication process.

Lack of access to CPOE resulted in delayed medication of patients. Unstable running of the CPOE system, lack of access to a computer, and staff without a system password were the immediate causes.

Finally, unstable data transfer between the patient administration system and the CPOE system has also been seen to cause delays in the medication process.

3.2. Complex User Interface

The user interface of the CPOE system has an intricate design which correlates with the complexity of the medication process itself. There are various examples of complex registration that lead to medication errors.

Examples of patient safety incidents are prescribing a drug for administration at the wrong date or time. The occasional need to scroll to see all prescriptions makes it difficult to maintain an overview.

Furthermore, important information can be “hiding” in a tool tip box or on a different screen page as the case is for all intravenous drug infusions (often antibiotics). This has resulted in overlooked prescriptions with the latter scenario having caused serious infections not to be appropriately treated for days. The issue relates to a certain design that was introduced to solve yet other registration problems.

An older, but still used version of the CPOE system poses problems regarding the registration of drug allergies: Due to the drug coding system in Denmark, when using this older version of the system, there is no simple way to secure that all administration formulas of a specific drug are covered when a drug allergy is registered. The reason for this is that the registration of an allergy is based on the ATC code, and the same drug can be registered under several codes if the drug has various indications.

The same problem exists regarding double medication (i.e. when the same or a similar drug is unintentionally prescribed twice). The older version of the CPOE system only warns the user if the same drug code appears twice and not if the same drug (registered under different ATC codes) appears twice.

3.3. Severe Errors Easily Made

The design of the CPOE system allows for errors such as order of magnitude errors (dosing times 10 or more) and unit errors (ml mistaken for IE for example) without providing a warning. Furthermore, when prescribing a drug in the CPOE system the route of administration is listed alphabetically and entered in by default (i.e. not left blank for the user to fill in). This has led to patient safety incidents where the default route of administration has not actively been changed to the intended route of administration by the doctor when prescribing a drug. Drugs for intravenous use have thus (unintentionally) been prescribed for epidural use, and potassium chloride for oral use has been administered intravenously - a potentially fatal incident.

4. Conclusion

The CPOE system is continuously being updated. Before implementing new design or functionality it is important to make a thorough risk assessment to ensure that the planned change will not introduce new risks.

Basic user education in the usage of the CPOE system is important. However, the reported patient safety incidents indicate that user education itself will not solve all problems.

In order to reduce the number of patient safety incidents it is important to take the "human factor" into consideration when designing a system like CPOE. Staff are prone to forget, misread, miswrite, over-look, and become interrupted. Alarming the user before executing a serious mistake is necessary, but the threshold for alarming must be carefully determined since an overload of alarms will reduce the likelihood of the user reacting appropriately. A well designed CPOE system should be intuitive, provide barriers against serious mistakes, and make the correct choice an easy one. Finally, it is important that the CPOE system closely supports the accepted clinical work routines.

References

The full report has been sent to The Danish National Board of Health on May 13, 2009 for display on their website.

Part C

Human Factors and Adverse Drug Events

Detection and Prevention of Adverse Drug Events
R. Beuscart et al. (Eds.)
IOS Press, 2009

doi:10.3233/978-1-60750-043-8-165

CPOE, Alerts and Workflow: Taking Stock of Ten Years Research at Erasmus MC

Jos AARTS, PhD [a,1] and Heleen VAN DER SIJS, MSc, RPh [b]
[a] *Institute of Health Policy and Management*
[b] *Department of Hospital Pharmacy, Erasmus MC, Rotterdam, The Netherlands*

Abstract. Ten years ago research of the impact of health information technology (HIT) on medical work practices started at Erasmus MC. The research is characterized by practice driven field research. From the beginning computerized physician order entry systems (CPOE) were a major topic. Research questions were how implementation of CPOE could be understood, how physicians were responding to reminders and alerts and how CPOE impacted professional workflow and collaboration. Studies of CPOE implementation aimed to understand why the adoption rate is so low and riddled with difficulties. Studies of reminders and alerts addressed the problem of alert fatigue. Finally, studies of workflow explored how CPOE influenced clinical workflow and how simplistic and linear models underlying CPOE may lead to poor designed systems and even compromise patient safety. Findings include the need for a shared understanding of medical challenges when implementing CPOE, conceptual models to understand alert fatigue and medical workflow and the impossibility of agreeing which alerts to suppress hospital-wide. The underlying research principle is the sociotechnical approach, which stipulates that technology, people and organizations should be studied from a single theoretical framework. This paper summarizes the results of ten years of research.

Keywords. Computerized physician order entry, Sociotechnical understanding, Impact on clinical work practices, Quantitaive and qualitive research, Field research

Introduction

Field studies have become important to understand the impact of health information technology on professionals and organizations. Field studies are characterized by observing use of information systems in situ. The methods utilized vary and may include direct observation, interviewing, studying documentation and surveying with questionnaires. Because of the complex nature of technology there usually is little room for experimentation, though some control may be possible, for example by observing work practices before and after implementation of information technology. Analysis is not necessarily exclusively qualitative, but is primarily aimed at offering descriptions and explanations. Careful theoretical argumentation is essential for the interpretation of the study results. Field studies came to the foreground when Massaro published his study how the introduction of a CPOE system in an academic medical center changed traditional work practices and forced clinicians to adopt new practice routines [1]. Detailed studies by Berg [2] of health information technology in practice have shown that the electronic patient record is not just a passive, perhaps even neutral, piece of

[1] Corresponding Author: j.aarts@erasmusmc.nl

technology that serves as a repository for patient data, but plays an active role in managing patient trajectories. Human models and norms are embedded in health information technology. An electronic prescribing system is designed purposely for physicians and cannot be used by nurses who have no prescription authority. Such purpose of design may well clash with the real world of hospital prescribing, in which often blank prescription forms carrying the signature of a physician can be filled out by the nurse in order to respond to a patient need when a doctor is unavailable. Health information systems that do not take account of the “messy” world of health practices may lead to workarounds unintended by its designers [3]. The approach to understand health information technology intertwined with its context of use is commonly known as the sociotechnical approach. It is this approach that has informed research at Erasmus MC for the last ten years [4].

1. Computerized Physician Order Entry Systems in the Netherlands

Computerized order entry (CPOE) systems allow clinicians to enter medications and other orders into a central electronic system. Those orders can be conveyed to a nurse station, pharmacy or other departments. CPOE systems have been introduced in the Netherlands since the early 1990s. Electronic prescribing has been widely adopted in primary care, though orders are not always conveyed to a public pharmacy to dispense medications to patients, but appear in print for a patient to take to the pharmacy [5]. Aarts et al. have conducted from 1999 until 2003 a longitudinal study of implementing CPOE in two Dutch hospitals. The implementation of CPOE in an academic medical center resulted in failure [6]. The researchers found that the reason to introduce electronic CPOE was not well articulated and communicated in the organization. The doctors considered the system primarily as an administrative burden. The situation became even more complicated when the system proved to be very cumbersome in use and slowed down administrative work processes. The CPOE system in the other hospital, a large regional medical center, became eventually a success because the nurses appreciated the value of electronic prescribing and documentation and therefore carried through the implementation in its most difficult period of acceptance [7]. Current physician usage in this hospital is estimated at 80%.

CPOE implementation in other academic medical centers started as pilots to improve medication prescribing for patients with complicated morbidity. Because pharmacists in Dutch hospitals were co-responsible for proper prescribing they became instrumental in the adoption of CPOE in Dutch hospitals. iSoft, a major vendor of hospital information systems in Dutch academic medical centers, developed in close collaboration with pharmacists a computerized physician medication order entry system [8]. The system, Medicatie/EVS, is currently being used in six academic medical centers, including Erasmus MC. A key component of the system is a decision support system that contains a drug-drug interaction database. The database, designed and maintained by the Royal Dutch Association for the Advancement of Pharmacy generates dedicated alert texts, which among others contains information for drug safety alerting for overdoses, duplicate orders and drug-drug interactions. The text also includes information on clinical consequences, mechanism and literature references. The database is seen as a professional standard for proper pharmaceutical care and has therefore been adopted nation-wide in primary, community pharmacies and hospitals [9]. In a recent study of CPOE in seven western countries Aarts and Koppel found that despite the recommendations of the Institute of Medicine uptake of CPOE systems is generally low, but that the Netherlands is ahead of the United States in CPOE use [10]. This fact went largely unnoticed in the international literature.

2. CPOE Research in Erasmus MC

Medicatie/EVS was introduced in Erasmus MC in December 2001, and in March 2005 all inpatient wards were using the system, except for the intensive care units, which use a patient data management system. Erasmus MC in Rotterdam, the Netherlands, comprises a 1,237-bed academic medical center consisting of three hospitals, a 800-bed general hospital, a children's hospital and an oncology clinic. The second author as a project leader for the implementation of Medicatie/EVS had been confronted with many complaints from physicians about annoying alerts generated by the system. The physicians asked whether these alerts could be turned off. She decided that quantitative research would probably not be sufficient to understand the nature of the problem and consulted in 2003 with Marc Berg, then professor at Erasmus MC, and the first author to discuss the problem at hand. She initiated a systematic study of alert overriding. At about the same time two Iranian medical doctors arrived to start a PhD study funded by their government. The authors assigned them to look at problems of the impact of health information technology on professional communication and medical workflow respectively. Though it was not planned as such, the presence of the CPOE system in Erasmus MC proved to be a fertile ground for these studies. The studies were grounded in the sociotechnical approach of clinical information systems described by Berg, Aarts and van der Lei [4], but quantitative data collection and analyses were equally part and parcel of the research methods. Field research also at Erasmus MC depends on observations, interviews, surveys and document studies. To a limited extent experiments were conducted to elicit responses, opinions and ideas of respondents.

The study of CPOE alerts started with a systematic review of drug safety alert overriding studies. Van der Sijs et al. found that in 49% to 96% of cases alerts were overridden [11]. They carefully analyzed the factors that play a role in overriding and proposed a model to understand the effect of overriding drug safety on patient safety based on Reason's model of accident causation. They emphasized that only unjustified overriding poses a problem. The authors argued that a safe alerting system has high specificity and sensitivity, presents clear information, does not unnecessarily disrupt workflow and facilitates safe and efficient handling. The authors suggested that improving alerting should focus on the prevention of active failures and individual error-producing conditions. Such a strategy would include reducing the number of inappropriate alerts, increasing sensitivity and usefulness and improve usability to disrupt workflow as little as possible. In an empirical study Van der Sijs et al. tried to answer the question whether frequently overridden drug alerts could be turned off safely [12]. The authors identified 24 frequently overridden alerts that accounted for 72% of all overridden drug-drug interaction alerts. Twenty-four clinicians evaluated these alerts. They reported that the main reasons for suppressing the alerts were "alert well known', "alert not serious or "alert not needing action." They also mentioned that effects of drug combinations were monitored or even intended. There was no agreement what alerts could be suppressed safely hospital-wide. In a simulation study to see whether in the adjusted drug-drug interaction database fewer alerts would be generated for a specific condition that would predispose patients for Torsades de

Pointes – a potential life-threatening arrhythmia – van der Sijs and her colleagues found that less patients at risk would be identified [13]. The adjustment did not clearly improve the identification of patients at risks and the authors suggested to maintain the old level of alerting and making more often an EKG, which would allow collecting more data to make a clinical rule that would result in more specific signaling.

CPOE systems have primarily been designed with the tasks and responsibilities of individual professionals in mind [14]. The models underlying CPOE systems tend to conceptualize order creation and communication as a pre-defined linear, linear and stepwise process, and fail to recognize the highly cognitive, collective, collaborative and ad hoc nature of clinical workflow. As part of her doctoral study of the impact of CPOE on clinical workflow Niazkhani and her colleagues conducted a systematic literature review study, in which they defined workflow as the allocation of multiple tasks of provider or of co-working providers in the processes of care and the way they collaborate [15]. They found that the impact of CPOE was double-edged. The review showed that CPOE resolved many disadvantages of workflow in paper-based practices, which include legibility and completeness of orders, availability of decision support and order sets, remote accessibility, possibility to view patient data simultaneously with other providers, and fewer interruptions. On the other hand the review revealed difficulties in workflow because of changes in the structure of work. Negative effects include cumbersome and time-consuming user-system interaction, the removal of important visual clues in paper-based systems, the enforcing of predefined and linear sequence of activities as well as a change of role-based relationships between professionals, synchronization of interdependent tasks and restrictions for team-based discussions. Niazkhani and her colleagues then tested their theoretical findings empirically, and based on available pre-and post-implementation data examined how nurses using two different paper-based medication prescribing and administration systems perceived the impact of Medicatie/EVS on their medication-related activities [16]. The two paper-based systems were different; the structure of nursing tasks in the system that used order forms, a.k.a. the Kardex system, was very similar to that of the CPOE system, but was different in the other system that allowed the physician to write down in free text a complete order. The nurses using the Kardex system reported a greater satisfaction with the CPOE system than the nurses using the other system. The differences could be explained be explained by the latter group's larger differences in work structure before and after implementation and a more difficult transition to CPOE. Analyzing the same pre- and post implementation data for six internal medicine wards combined with interviews Pirnejad et al. found how Medicatie/EVS disrupted nurse-physician communication in the medication administration process and suggested improvements in the design making nurses responsible for printing prescription orders [17].

3. Conclusion

We have presented in this paper CPOE research conducted at Erasmus MC in the last decade. To a considerable part this research has been informed by the sociotechnical approach to understand the intertwinement of technology and clinical context. Studying systems in practice imposes limitations to the researcher because opportunities to 'experiment' and control variables are limited. However, field research offers the opportunity to study systems in real use. We found for example that there are limited opportunities to turn off frequently overridden alerts hospital-wide and that more tailored approaches are necessary. Our research still left many questions open, especially about physician behavior when dealing with alerts. Our results may help inform better design and implementation practices. One of the results of our research efforts has been the establishment of a research group as collaboration between the departments of Hospital Pharmacy and Medical Informatics and the Institute of Health Policy and Management of Erasmus MC to study the interrelationship between medication safety and health information technology. Research challenges include electronic prescribing across organizational boundaries, electronic medication administration records and administration errors, cognitive understanding of alert overriding and the development of an observational database of electronic ordering, alert generation and overrides, and medication administration.

References

[1] Massaro TA. Introducing physician order entry at a major academic medical center: I. Impact on organizational culture and behavior. Acad Med. 1993 Jan;68(1):20-5.
[2] Berg M, Goorman E. The contextual nature of medical information. Int J Med Inform. 1999 Dec;56(1-3):51-60.
[3] Goorman E, Berg M. Modelling nursing activities: electronic patient records and their discontents. Nurs Inq. 2000 Mar;7(1):3-9.
[4] Berg M, Aarts J, Van Der Lei J. ICT in health care: sociotechnical approaches. Methods Inf Med. 2003;42(4):297-301.
[5] Schoen C, Osborn R, Huynh PT, Doty M, Peugh J, Zapert K. On the front lines of care: primary care doctors' office systems, experiences, and views in seven countries. Health Aff (Millwood). 2006 Nov-Dec;25(6):w555-71.
[6] Aarts J, Doorewaard H, Berg M. Understanding implementation: the case of a computerized physician order entry system in a large Dutch university medical center. J Am Med Inform Assoc. 2004 May-Jun;11(3):207-16.
[7] Aarts J, Berg M. Same systems, different outcomes - comparing the implementation of computerized physician order entry in two Dutch hospitals. Methods Inf Med. 2006;45(1):53-61.
[8] Kalmeijer MD, Holtzer W, van Dongen R, Guchelaar HJ. Implementation of a computerized physician medication order entry system at the Academic Medical Centre in Amsterdam. Pharm World Sci. 2003 Jun;25(3):88-93.
[9] van Roon EN, Flikweert S, le Comte M, Langendijk PN, Kwee-Zuiderwijk WJ, Smits P, et al. Clinical relevance of drug-drug interactions : a structured assessment procedure. Drug Saf. 2005;28(12):1131-9.
[10] Aarts J, Koppel R. Implementation of computerized physician order entry in seven countries. Health Aff (Millwood). 2009 Mar-Apr;28(2):404-14.
[11] van der Sijs H, Aarts J, Vulto A, Berg M. Overriding of drug safety alerts in computerized physician order entry. J Am Med Inform Assoc. 2006 Mar-Apr;13(2):138-47.
[12] van der Sijs H, Aarts J, van Gelder T, Berg M, Vulto A. Turning off frequently overridden drug alerts: limited opportunities for doing it safely. J Am Med Inform Assoc. 2008 Jul-Aug;15(4):439-48.
[13] van der Sijs H, Kowlesar R, Aarts J, Berg M, Vulto A, van Gelder T. Unintended consequences of reducing QT-alert overload in a computerized physician order entry system. Eur J Clin Pharmacol. 2009 May 5.
[14] Aarts J, Ash J, Berg M. Extending the understanding of computerized physician order entry: Implications for professional collaboration, workflow and quality of care. Int J Med Inform. 2007 Jun;76 Suppl 1:4-13.
[15] Niazkhani Z, Pirnejad H, Berg M, Aarts J. The impact of computerized provider order entry (CPOE) systems on inpatient clinical workflow: a literature review. J Am Med Inform Assoc. 2009 Apr 23.
[16] Niazkhani Z, van der Sijs H, Pirnejad H, Redekop WK, Aarts J. Same system, different outcomes: comparing the transitions from two paper-based systems to the same computerized physician order entry system. Int J Med Inform. 2009 Mar;78(3):170-81.
[17] Pirnejad H, Niazkhani Z, van der Sijs H, Berg M, Bal R. Impact of a computerized physician order entry system on nurse-physician collaboration in the medication process. Int J Med Inform. 2008 Nov;77(11):735-44.

Detection and Prevention of Adverse Drug Events
R. Beuscart et al. (Eds.)
IOS Press, 2009

doi:10.3233/978-1-60750-043-8-170

Contribution of Human Factors for the Review of Automatically Detected ADE

Nicolas LEROY [a,1], Michel LUYCKX [b], Philippe LECOCQ [b], Romaric MARCILLY [a] and Marie-Catherine BEUSCART-ZÉPHIR [a]

[a] *Univ Lille Nord de France; INSERM CIC-IT-Evalab, Lille; CHU Lille; UDSL EA 2694; F-59000 Lille, France*

[b] *Centre Hospitalier de Denain, F- 59220 France; faculte de pharmacie, Univ Lille Nord de France, F-59000 Lille, France*

Abstract. The European project PSIP (Patient Safety through Intelligent Procedures in Medication) aims at semi-automatically identifying and preventing ADE. Automatically detected Adverse Drug Events have to be reviewed and validated by human experts. Existing methods usually have the experts review the cases and document their rating in a structured form. One of the limitations of these methods is their poor ability to analyze and clear the disagreements between the experts and the system. This paper presents an innovative Human Factors based method to support the review by clinicians and pharmacologists of these automatically detected ADE. We use think aloud methods and portable labs to track and record the experts reasoning and their reviewing cognitive procedures. We present preliminary results obtained with this method, which allows identifying the key data and information used to characterize the ADE. This method provides useful feedbacks allowing a continuous refinement and improvement of the automated detection system.

Keywords. Adverse Drug Event (ADE), Knowledge Elicitation, Think Aloud protocols, cognitive processes

Introduction

In the last decade, Adverse Drug Events (ADE) due to medication errors and human factors have progressively been considered a major public health issue. ADE endanger the patients' safety and cause considerable extra healthcare costs [1]. Most authors adopt the rather general definition of ADE provided by the IOM: "an injury caused by medical management rather than the underlying condition of a patient" [1]. ADE may be the result of an unexpected Adverse Drug Reaction (ADR) or of a medication error defined as "the failure of a planned action to be completed as intended of the use of a wrong plan to achieve an aim" [1;2].

Improving patient safety through a significant diminution of ADE requires a twofold process. It is first necessary to know the epidemiology and the nature of Adverse Drug Events, i.e. their prevalence, medical characteristics, context of occurrence etc. Usual methods to accomplish this goal are mainly retrospective analyses of medical records or of ADE cases reported in specific reporting systems

[1] Corresponding Author: Nicolas LEROY, Evalab, Faculté de Médecine, 1 Place de Verdun, 59000 Lille, France - nicolas.leroy-2@univ-lille2.fr

dedicated to medical Adverse Events or Incidents. Secondly it is necessary to change the work system to prevent potential future ADE to occur. The knowledge gathered in the first step allows prospectively identifying dangerous healthcare situations where a risk of ADE is highly probable. Relying on the ADE characteristics identified in the retrospective phase, efficient counter measures can be implemented. One of the possible forms of counter measure is the delivery to healthcare professionals of contextualized knowledge focused on the problem such as Decision Support Systems.

The ever increasing availability of large repositories of patients' medical data constituted from Electronic Health Records (EHR), Hospital / Clinical Information Systems (HIS, CIS) provides the researchers the opportunity to develop innovative tools able to (i) semi-automatically search retrospectively these medical repositories to identify potential ADE (ii) prospectively identify the dangerous situations to deliver the healthcare professionals a contextual knowledge aiming at preventing the ADE[3-6].

In such projects, it is necessary to have human experts validate the results automatically provided by screening or mining techniques. Moreover, the qualitative feedbacks collected through the analysis of the reviewers' results may efficiently support the continuous refinement of the mining procedures. This paper presents the Human Factors supported methods used in PSIP to perform this validation.

1. Background and Context

1.1. The PSIP Strategy to Identify and Prevent ADE

PSIP addresses the problem of ADE detection by searching large repositories of electronic medical records and data in order to detect abnormal cases presenting typical ADE features [7]. Data mining techniques performed on these medical data allow identifying "abnormal" hospital stays (i.e. suspect of an ADE) along with the association rules statistically linked with these stays [7]. An example of rule issued by a decision tree is "*If nutrient and Proton Pump Inhibitor and age>80 ➔ risk of hyponatremia*". For each context a rule is characterized by:

- its confidence i.e. the number of positive cases for the predictor
- its support, i.e. the number of positive cases vs the number of cases matching the conditions

For the above mentioned rule, in one medical unit of the French Denain hospital 8 stays match the predictor (conditions of the rule) and 7 present the effect "hyponatremia" (confidence = 7/8 = 87%, support = 7).

These association rules constitute the basic knowledge that is to be implemented in the PSIP Computer Supported Decision System (CDSS). This CDSS prospectively identifies similar dangerous cases (same conditions) and delivers the healthcare professionals an ad hoc knowledge helping them to prevent the effect or ADE to occur.

1.2. Validation of Data Mining Results by Human Experts

When records pointing at a potential ADE are retrospectively automatically identified, it is mandatory that human experts review a sample of normal/abnormal cases to validate their characterization as "normal" vs. "potential ADE" and the clinical relevance of this automatic categorization [4;8;9]. In this approach, the experts' judgment is considered a gold standard.

Moreover, in complex projects like PSIP, it is critical that the expert reviewers validate the clinical relevance of the rules associated with an abnormal stay: once implemented in the CDS system, the premises of the rule will identify suspect cases of potential ADE and correspondingly the system will deliver the clinicians the knowledge incorporated in the rule. Thus validating the clinical relevance of the rule when considering the cases they have targeted as ADE is critical to ensure the upcoming efficiency and acceptance of the PSIP CDSS modules.

Other authors have described methods to support the experts' review and validation of electronically screened medical records [9-11]. Judgments concerning ADEs are supported by structured data forms such as the Adverse Event Analysis form developed by investigators in the Harvard Medical Practice Study (MPS) [12]. This method allows categorizing the corresponding cases as actual ADE or not. It then allows calculating an inter-experts agreement and the accuracy of the automatic detection of ADE (True / False Positives / Negatives). However, the method also presents some limitations, the most important one being that this manual review process is time consuming. Moreover, although the structured data form gives the experts the opportunity to characterize the validated ADEs on a number of variables, it does not provide enough information on the experts reasoning to analyze the reasons why the experts disagreed (or agreed) with each other and/or with the automatic categorization of the cases as ADE / Non ADE.

In the PSIP project, we try to circumvent these limitations and to take a step further. We take advantage of the existence of the common data model and of the availability of all the clinical data in a common repository to use a web-based query application specifically developed by one of the PSIP partners. This application, the Expert Explorer® gives the reviewers access to all the data of a given case. Moreover, the application also includes an automated version of the questionnaire supporting the experts' judgment. Thus the reviewing tasks may be performed on-line. We use Human Factors techniques and methods such as Think Aloud protocols and portable usability labs to monitor and record the experts' activities (behavioral and cognitive ones) while reviewing the cases and assessing the corresponding rules. The main objective is to understand the experts' reasoning and to identify the parameters or data they rely on to interpret and validate / invalidate both the ADE cases and the clinical relevance of the association rule attached to the stay in order to provide useful feedbacks for the data mining procedures.

2. Methods

2.1. The Validation Procedure

The expert review method is divided into three main steps described in Figure 1.

4. During the first step of the review process, the expert logs in the Expert Explorer and accesses his pending list of stays to review. The selection of a stay allows him to navigate freely through all the data of this stay. No order of visualization is imposed.
5. When the expert is done with the reading and analysis of the data, he can move on the second step i.e. the characterization of the case in terms of ADE /

non ADE. This characterization is supported by a structured form adapted from the Adverse Event Analysis form developed by the investigators in the Harvard Medical Practice Study [12]. In the PSIP version, once an expert has identified a preventable ADE, he can select from the list displayed by the Expert Explorer the drugs and/or the lab results of the stay he thinks are connected to the ADE.

6. Whether the expert has characterized the stay under review as "ADE" or "NO ADE" in the second step, if this stay is characterized as "Abnormal" by the data mining, the corresponding association rule is presented to the reviewer in the third and last step of the review. The expert is then asked to assess the validity of the rule in general and in the specific clinical context of the case.

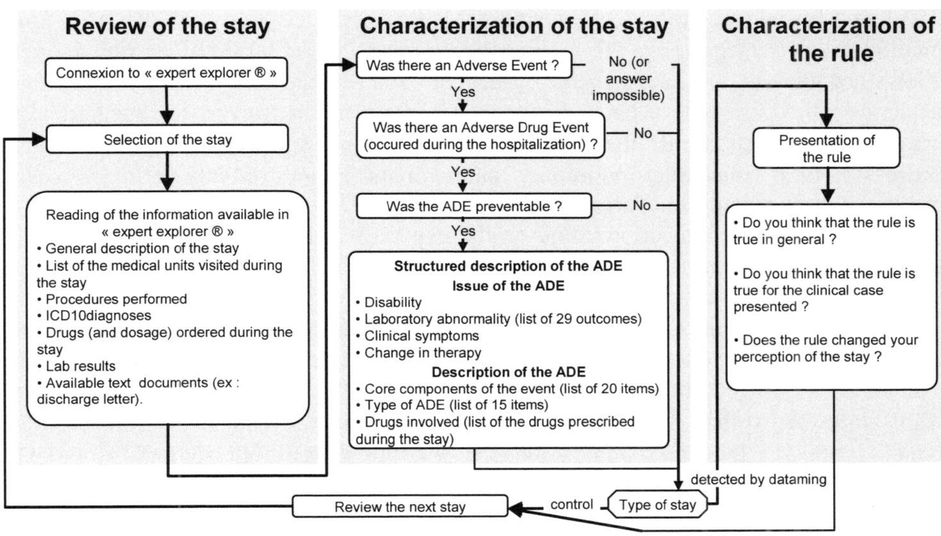

Figure 1 General description of the Expert review process (see the text for details)

2.2. Material and Subjects

2445 hospitalization stays have been exported from the Denain hospital medical units in the common database. About 40 rules issued from the decision trees run on these 2445 stays were available at the time of the study. We selected at random 14 rules. Altogether these 14 rules targeted 121 stays matching the conditions and showing the negative effects or probable ADE. We selected at random again 43 cases among these 121 "abnormal" stays. Those 43 abnormal cases were mixed with 37 "normal" stays, selected at random from all the stays showing none of the effects defined in the data model, thus providing a final sample of 80 cases to be reviewed.

Across all the steps of the reviewing process, the Experts are asked to "think aloud" Their verbalizations are recorded along with their actions with the "Expert Explorer ®". The technical apparatus used for the recording incorporates a microphone and a PC connected to the Internet allowing accessing to the "Expert Explorer®" viewer application. "The Camtasia 5®" software is used to record both Experts' actions and verbalizations.

2.3. Method for the Analysis of Video / Verbal Protocols

The Morae® software is used to analyze the videos and to divide them into meaningful behavioral units, depending on the stage of the review process, the data reviewed, the item of the questionnaire under consideration etc. In parallel, the experts' verbalizations are typewritten and divided into corresponding semantic units. Excerpts of the protocols may then be coded according to a specific coding scheme aiming for example at identifying the root causes of inter-experts disagreements about the clinical relevance of the rule. The coding of the semantic units is performed blindly by two authors (NL & RM). At the end of the coding, a debriefing phase allows the authors (1) reaching a consensus on potential disagreements in their initial coding of the semantic units and (2) refining the coding grid.

3. Results

The reviewing process of the 80 cases of the Denain hospital is currently under progress. We present here preliminary results obtained on a sub-sample of 53 cases mixing 32 "abnormal" cases with 21 "control" cases.

3.1. General Description of the Categorization of the Stays

Table 1 displays an overview of experts and data-mining agreement on cases categorization. The experts' concordance for the characterization of the stays is 35/53 (66 %) with a κ score of 0,32 (κ/κmax=.38). For 30 of those stays (56,6%), both experts also agree with the data mining characterization. Independently each expert's concordance with the data mining is 38/53 (72%). For 43 stays out of 53 (81%) there is at least one expert agreeing with the data mining characterization. For five stays (9,4%), there is one expert selecting the "Answer impossible" option due to a lack of information.

Table 1: Distribution of the characterization of the 53 cases according to expert1-expert2 agreement and experts-data mining (DM) agreement – κ=.36 (κ/κmax =.38).

			expert 2			
			agree with the DM characterization	disagree with the DM characterization	Answer impossible	Total
expert 1	agree with the DM characterization	nb	30	8	0	38
		%	56,6%	15,1%	0,0%	71,7%
	disagree with the DM characterization	nb	5	5	1	11
		%	9,4%	9,4%	1,9%	20,8%
	Answer impossible	nb	3	1	0	4
		%	5,7%	1,9%	0,0%	7,5%
	Total	nb	38	14	1	53
		%	71,7%	26,4%	1,9%	100,0%

3.2. Inter Experts and Experts-DM Agreement on Detection of ADEs

Both experts agree with the DM characterization of the "control" stays as "No ADE" for all 21 cases. The expert-expert concordance and the experts-DM concordance are therefore maximal (100%). Two ADE occurring before the hospitalization are detected by the experts from the discharge letter but this category of ADE is outside the current PSIP scope.

Concerning the 32 DM abnormal stays, 10 stays (31%) are characterized as actual ADE by both experts and 15 (47 %) are characterized as ADE by only one of them (**Figure**). All in all, 78% of abnormal stays detected by PSIP are considered as ADE by at least one of the two experts.

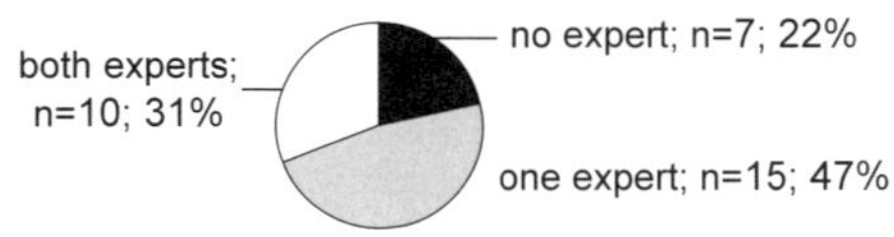

Figure 2. Experts' categorization of the 32 PSIP "abnormal" stays as actual ADE

3.3. Validation of the ADEs' Outcomes

The abnormal cases submitted to the experts for review often correspond to complex and long hospital stays. Then it may happen that the experts identify another ADE than the one targeted by the rule. The questionnaire filled by the experts in the "characterization of the stay" stage of the review allows to confront the ADE or outcome spontaneously identified by the experts with the one identified by PSIP.

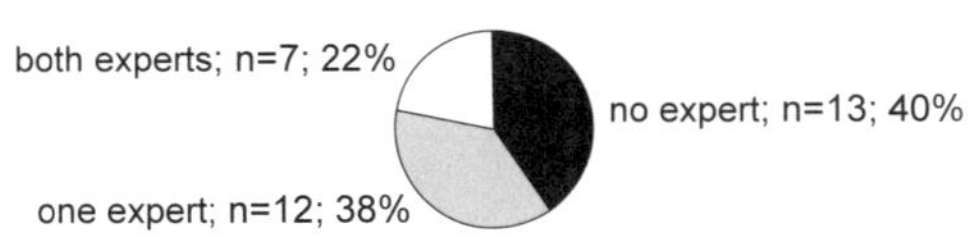

Figure 3. Distribution of DM-experts agreement concerning the identification of the outcomes targeted by PSIP and validated by none, one or both Experts

Both experts validate the outcome targeted by PSIP for 7 stays (22 %) and 12 stays (38 %) are validated by only one expert as illustrated in **Figure** . All in all, 60% of the negative outcomes identified by PSIP are spontaneously validated by at least one of the two experts.

3.4. Validation of the Rule in the Clinical Context

Both experts validate the PSIP rule for 4 abnormal stays (13 %) and at least one of the experts validates the rule for 8 stays (25 %). All in all, the PSIP rules are validated for the stays under review by only one expert in 38% of the cases. But this leaves 28 stays out of the 32 targeted by the different PSIP rules for which at least one expert rejects the rule for the case under review. It has to be noted that Expert 1 uses the answer "do not know" 4 times (12 %) while the Expert 2 uses it 9 times (28 %), which shows the difficulty of the question.

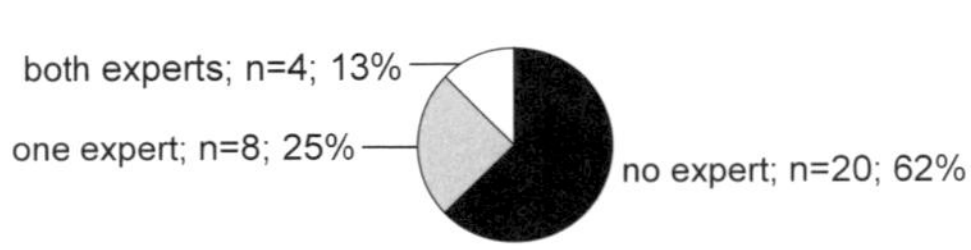

Figure 4. Number and percentage of rules validated in the clinical context of the stay by none, one or both experts

3.5. Qualitative Analysis of the Experts' Decision Making

3.5.1. Analysis of the Experts' Decision Making Pathways

Figure 5 displays the type of sequences of decisions taken by both experts at each step of the reviewing process for the 32 abnormal cases. The combinations of the successive steps issue 11 different categories of final decisions on the stay and on the clinical relevance of the PSIP rule.

Interestingly, the figure shows that an expert may initially select another ADE than the one identified in PSIP or even decide that a stay is not an ADE and then change his mind when presented with the PSIP rule (category d), ultimately deciding that the rule makes sense and explains the case at hand (category d). In those cases the PSIP rule brings the experts a knowledge that was not readily available to them.

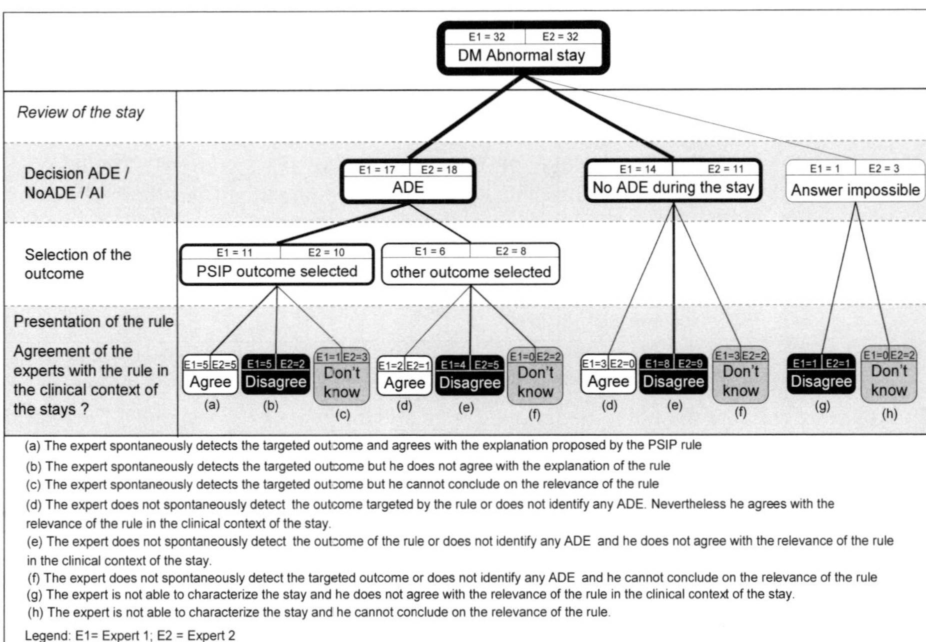

Figure 5. Expert' decision making pathways when performing the review of the 32 DM-abnormal stays

3.5.2. Analysis of Experts' Justifications of their Decision Making

We performed a detailed analysis of experts' verbalizations while filling the last part of the questionnaire (characterization of the rule) for all categories but "a" and "d" (see figure 5). The objective of this analysis was to identify the experts' justification for not agreeing with the PSIP rule attached to the stays under review. We designed a coding scheme in order to categorize the levels and reasons for disagreement. This coding scheme identifies three main levels of experts-DM disagreement: the experts may have problems with the data, or with the information derived from these data (i.e. interpreted data), or with the relationship established by PSIP between the causes and the outcome of the ADE. Regarding the data level, experts may think that they are corrupted (technical problem = A) or inexplicably missing (B). Regarding the Information level, experts may doubt the threshold level of abnormality independently of the clinical context (C) or they question the medical judgment on the data in the clinical context (D), mostly because these data are explained by other characteristics of the patients' case. Finally, at the rule level the experts usually argue that the rule maybe true but not applicable in the clinical context at hand (E).

45 verbalizations have been analyzed and coded, 19 from expert 1 and 26 from expert 2. These verbalizations concern the 28 stays for which at least one expert have rejected the PSIP rule (see fig.4). Table 2 displays the main results of the coding and the number of stays, out of the 28 above mentioned, to which each category of explanation applies. For each stay, experts may express different types of disagreement, in average 2.21. For the most complicate stay, six different explanations were provided.

Table 2. Categories and examples of coded semantic units accounting for experts-DM disagreements on the relevance of the PSIP rule in the clinical context of the stay targeted by the rule and number of stays concerned by the explanation

Levels of disagreemen t	Type of problems		sub-class		Number of stays (out of the 28)	example of units of meaning
Data	Technical problems with data	A	A1	incomplete data about outcome	1	"platelets, yes, but the first part of the stay is missing »"
	Incomplete clinical data	B	B1	lack of data about the outcome	5	"Can't say, I don't have the admission lab results"
			B2	lack of data about the cause	4	"we don't have access to the home treatment "
Information	Problems with thresholds of the parameters used in the rules outside the clinical context	C	C1	threshold of detection of the outcomes	**10**	"Yes, but it is a very very tiny effect, it's just over the superior bound"
			C2	threshold of detection of the causes	5	"the drug has been only administrated the first day. I cant trust it, not for only one day"
	Problems with the judgment on the data in the clinical context	D	D1	data explained by patients' characteristics	**9**	"Dying patients have a lot of health problems"
			D2	Normal patient's' reaction to his/her treatment	1	"No, because the thrombocytopenia is due to the chemotherapy »"
			D3	outcome caused by another cause	7	" I think that the hyponatremia is due to the glucose solution"

Relation Cause-Outcome of the rule	Rule not true in the context	E	E1	Rule not applicable (problems with administration route and chronology)	**16**	"the thrombocytosis appears on day 17 while the metronidazole treatment is given on days 1, 2 and 3, so the delay is too important" «oral antifungic : it can't go through the digestive system. So we can't find it in the blood. It can't impact the lab results. »
			E2	Rule not applicable, effect disappears without change in the drugs' administration)	4	"The treatment is neither modified nor suspended and it goes back to normal on its own, urea, creatinin, so for me, it's not the drug"

The most frequent explanations (category E1, 16/28 stays) are related to problems of rules' application e.g. the drug could provoke this outcome but not by that route of administration, or the delay between the drug administration and the appearance of the effect is too long. The second most frequent explanation (C1, 10/28) refers to problems of threshold of detection of the outcome in the lab results, the experts doubting the effect because the lab value is not "abnormal" enough. Almost equally frequent are the explanations referring to patients' characteristics as probable "other" cause (D1, 9/28) of the observed outcome or ADE. Conversely, technical problems such as inexplicably missing data are rare.

4. Discussion and Conclusion

In this study the concordance between the experts' judgments is moderate to low, with a κ index <.40. Some studies using the MPS Adverse Event Analysis form in Medical Chart Review tasks have found similar concordance with a κ index ranging in the .40 [8;13]. But in most of the studies the experts are trained beforehand and the results consequently show a better concordance [10]. However in the present study we are mostly interested in the experts' qualitative feedbacks on the causality of the ADE and the clinical relevance of the rules. Therefore, formatting the experts' strategies and answer is not of primary interest in this first iteration of the review process.

In spite of the limitation of the low inter-experts agreement, each expert's categorization of the stays is relatively consistent with that of the data mining. There are no false negatives at all, and 78 % of the stays detected by the data mining procedure contained an ADE according to at least one of the experts. These results obtained with a first iteration of the data mining techniques are promising. The refinement of the data mining techniques following the qualitative feedbacks from the experts review should help continuously improve the accuracy of the ADE detection.

The outcomes or ADE identified by the experts do not always correspond to the one identified by the data mining. This may be due to the fact that the ADE stays may contain more than one ADE, as has been observed in other studies [10]. In this first iteration of the review process, the selection procedure of the sample of stays to be reviewed had identified only one rule per stay. The qualitative analysis of the experts' answers and comments will allow checking the ADE stays for other negative outcomes and verify whether the data mining procedures are able to catch those other outcomes.

The experts often disagreed with the data mining about the validity of the rule in the clinical context (18/32 for Expert 1 and 17/32 for Expert 2) or selected the "I don't know" box (4/32 for Expert 1 and 9/32 for Expert 2). The detailed analysis of the experts' verbal protocols allows categorizing and clarifying the reasons of these disagreements. These detailed results of the review process and particularly the experts' comments on the rule in the clinical context constitute valuable feedbacks for the partners in charge of the data model and of the data mining. Indeed some changes have already been implemented in the data mining procedures such as less strict thresholds for "abnormal" values. This intertwinement between the qualitative analysis of the review results and the data mining techniques supports a continuous improvement of the PSIP techniques for ADE detection.

Finally, the analysis of the reviewing experts' behavior and comments provide interesting clues for the user-centered design of the future PSIP CDSS modules. For instance the experts systematically confront the evolution of the lab results and more specifically any abrupt variations of these results with the modifications in the medication orders. They even try to trick the system in order to display both types of information simultaneously on the screen. Correspondingly, the CDSS module should display the recent evolution of relevant lab results at the time the physician is ordering the drug or remind him to monitor it when the lab values are missing.

In this first iteration of the review process, the most interesting results and feedbacks come from the analysis of the verbal/video protocols. Unfortunately, this analysis of video protocols is highly time-consuming. Therefore the method cannot be used in the long run. But from the results obtained in this first round, it is possible to adapt and extend the current questionnaire in order to catch specifically the information that is currently retrieved through the video analysis. The modified and extended questionnaire is currently under validation. It will then be implemented in the Expert Explorer© tool to support the ongoing review process. This should help continuously improving both the accuracy of ADE detection and the tuning of the PSIP CDSS modules.

Acknowledgement

The research leading to these results has received funding from the European Community's Seventh Framework Programme (FP7/2007-2013) under Grant Agreement n° 216130 - the PSIP project.

References

[1] Kohn LT, Corrigan J. M., and Donaldson M. S. To Err is Human. 1999. Washington, DC., National academy Press.
[2] Institute Of Medicine, Preventing Medication Errors. The National Academic Press, Washington, DC, 2007.
[3] Seger AC, Jha AK, and Bates DW, Adverse drug event detection in a community hospital utilising computerised medication and laboratory data. Drug Saf 30: 817-824, 2007.
[4] Morimoto T, Gandhi TK, Seger AC, Hsieh TC, and Bates DW, Adverse drug events and medication errors: detection and classification methods. Qual Saf Health Care 13: 306-314, 2004.
[5] Leroy N, Chazard E., Beuscart R., and Beuscart-Zephir MC, Toward automatic detection and prevention of adverse drug events. Stud Health Technol Inform 143: 30-35, 2009.
[6] Murff HJ, Patel VL, Hripcsak G, and Bates DW, Detecting adverse events for patient safety research: a review of current methodologies. J.Biomed.Inform 36: 131-143, 2003.
[7] Chazard E., Preda C., Merlin B., Ficheur G., and Beuscart R., Datamining based detection of adverse drug events. Stud Health Technol Inform In Press: 2009.
[8] Bates DW, Evans RS, Murff H, Stetson PD, Pizziferri L, and Hripcsak G, Detecting Adverse Drug Events using Information Technology. The Journal of the American Medical Informatics Association 10: 115-128, 2003.
[9] Murff HJ, Forster AJ, Peterson JF, Fiskio JM, Heiman HL, and Bates DW, Electronically screening discharge summaries for adverse medical events. J.Am.Med.Inform Assoc. 10: 339-350, 2003.
[10] Kilbridge PM, Campbell UC, Cozart HB, and Mojarrad MG, Automated surveillance for adverse drug events at a community hospital and an academic medical center. J.Am.Med.Inform Assoc. 13: 372-377, 2006.
[11] Jha AK, Laguette J, Seger A, and Bates DW, Can surveillance systems identify and avert adverse drug events? A prospective evaluation of a commercial application. J.Am.Med.Inform Assoc. 15: 647-653, 2008.
[12] Brennan TA, Leape LL, Laird NM, Hebert L, Localio AR, Lawthers AG, Newhouse JP, Weiler PC, and Hiatt HH, Incidence of adverse events and negligence in hospitalized patients. Results of the Harvard Medical Practice Study I. N.Engl.J.Med. 324: 370-376, 1991.
[13] Thomas EJ, Lipsitz SR, Studdert DM, and Brennan TA, The reliability of medical record review for estimating adverse event rates. Ann.Intern.Med. 136: 812-816, 2002.

Detection and Prevention of Adverse Drug Events
R. Beuscart et al. (Eds.)
IOS Press, 2009

doi:10.3233/978-1-60750-043-8-181

A Framework for Diagnosing and Identifying Where Technology-Induced Errors Come From

E. M. BORYCKI [a, 1], A. W. KUSHNIRUK [a], L. KEAY [a] and A. KUO [a]
[a]*School of Health Information Science, University of Victoria, Victoria, British Columbia, Canada*

Abstract. Health information systems have the ability to reduce medical errors but they can also introduce new types of errors. In the cognitive and human factors literature there is a recognition that many of the high profile accidents that have occurred in other industries outside of healthcare have had their origins in the complexities of organizational work and how work is structured. The authors propose that in order to have a fully robust framework for diagnosing technology-induced errors one must understand the development and implementation of a technology and the influences of policy using a multi-organizational model. The authors propose that technology-induced errors may have their origins in up to four or more organizational structures that make up complex health care systems in addition to the health care provider: governments, model organizations, software development organizations, and local healthcare organizations. In this paper a framework for considering the origins of technology-induced error in healthcare is presented, along with our experiences to date in the application of the framework.

Keywords. EPR-CPR-EMR, human interfaces, patient safety, technology-induced error, frameworks, health informatics, health information systems, organizational behaviour, complex systems

Introduction

Health information systems have the ability to reduce medical errors but they can also introduce new types of errors (i.e. technology-induced errors) to an existing complex or error prone healthcare system. Technology-induced errors are not a new phenomena in healthcare. One of the earliest documented reports of technology-induced errors in healthcare dates back to investigations conducted into the design, development and operation of Therac 25 – a device used to provide radiation therapy to cancer patients [1].

More recently, the ability of technology to introduce errors has emerged as an issue where electronic health records (EHRs) and their associated devices (e.g. workstations, wireless carts and palm devices) are concerned. Researchers in the health or biomedical informatics literature have begun to identify those types of errors that health information systems and their associated devices could introduce to the healthcare workplace (e.g. [2-3]). As a result researchers have begun to develop

[1] Corresponding Author: E. M. Borycki, E-mail: emb@uvic.ca

schemes to identify and classify these types of errors. Researchers have also begun to explore, develop and test new methodologies that can be used to identify or capture the occurrence of technology-induced errors at point of care (e.g. [2-4]).

Technology induced errors or "those types of errors that technologies can introduce or propagate" [5, p.153] are increasingly being attended to by the health informatics and quality improvement community. For example; the Joint Commission for Health Care Quality issued a sentinel events bulletin stating: "As health information technology (HIT) and 'converging technologies'—the interrelationship between medical devices and HIT—are increasingly adopted by health care organizations, users must be mindful of the safety risks and preventable adverse events that these implementations can create or perpetuate". Technology-related adverse events can be associated with all components of a comprehensive technology system and may involve errors of either commission or omission. These unintended adverse events typically stem from human-machine interfaces or organization/system design." [6, p.1]. Over the next few years as we move towards using health information systems and their associated devices to provide patient care, there will be a need to identify the sources of technology induced-errors so that we can prevent them from occurring. The purpose of this paper will be to describe a framework that draws on the work of Reason [7], Orlikowski [8], Borycki [5], Keay [14] and Kushniruk [3] and demonstrate its value in providing a comprehensive framework for identifying the possible sources of technology-induced errors in healthcare. The framework may be used as a tool to examine the organizational origin(s) of technology-induced errors and identify the organizational areas that need to be reviewed to prevent technology induced-error from occurring in the future.

1. Literature Review

In the cognitive and human factors literature there is a recognition that many of the high profile accidents that have occurred in other industries outside of healthcare (i.e. Three Mile Island and Chernobyl in the nuclear industry and aircraft accidents) [9] have had their origins in the complexities of organizational work and how work is structured [7,9]. In general researchers agree that the human that is involved in the error is only a "starting point" and that in order to fully understand how an error occurs there is a need to examine the organization and its processes to identify the source of the error and prevent it from occurring again [10]. This research is in keeping with the research and reports from leading researchers in the quality improvement literature who have suggested that 90% of the issues associated with the quality of a product or service (i.e. defects in either) have their origins in organizational processes rather than the individual worker being responsible for the error or defect [16].

Reason [7] has developed a model of error where he distinguishes between a "sharp end", which is where work is performed and individual errors may occur, and a "blunt end" where errors may arise from organizational complexity. According to Reason [7] most errors are made by humans at the sharp end, where work is undertaken by individuals, but they have their origins in the complex, organizational systems, processes and environments that are constructed by organizations in order for humans to perform their work (i.e. the blunt end of error) [7]. Therefore, when identifying the cause of an error one can begin by investigating the sharp end of the error and move towards the origin of the error at the blunt end to prevent the error from occurring and propagating through the through system to the sharp end [7, 10].

In the healthcare and more specifically in the health informatics literature there is a need to understand the potential root causes of technology-induced errors and to examine the constellations of policies, practices, processes and events that may lead to a technology-induced error occurring at the sharp end with the health care provider (e.g. physician or nurse). Research in the health informatics literature has for the most part focused on identifying the sharp end of technology-induced errors. This research has involved observing health professionals interacting with health information systems and their associated devices in real world settings after a health information system and its associated devices have been deployed in the clinical setting (e.g. [2,4]) as well as examining real-world occurrences of sharp end technology-induced errors after they have occurred as part of an investigation into their occurrence (e.g. [11]). In an effort to identify these potential causes of error, researchers have developed methods aimed at diagnosing error further away from the sharp, human end of technology-induced errors. The research has led to the application and development of methodological approaches that could be employed in diagnosing errors at the blunt end (i.e. before systems implementation) and before the error occurs at the sharp end. Researchers have applied methods from the fields of usability engineering [3,18], cognitive engineering [9, 12] and clinical simulation [15], identifying potential downstream technology-induced errors to prevent sharp end occurrences [13]. Recent research has been successful in identifying blunt end sources of errors in complex systems. Kushniruk et al. [3] was able to use usability testing techniques to identify user interface attributes that lead to increases in medication errors (e.g. the presence of medication dosage defaults) prior to systems implementation. In another study researchers used clinical simulations in conjunction with workflow mapping to identify potential sources of error arising from interactions between a device, health information system and the health care providers work environment prior to the device-system implementation [17]. Both of these studies suggested that blunt end sources of error (i.e. those arising from software development and implementation of systems and devices) contributed to sharp end error. Some researchers even began to explore the implications of presenting such blunt end work over time within the context of a health care system to better understand the system wide implications of not addressing these blunt end causes of errors at a health care system level [14].

This work when considered in conjunction with the work of Reason [7] and Vincente [9], suggests there is even more reason to explore the blunt causes of technology-induced error in health care. A framework that attempts to understand the blunt end causes of technology-induced error was proposed by Keay and Kushniruk [14]. The researchers attempted to identify the possible blunt end causes of technology-induced errors involving health information systems and their devices. Borycki and Kushniruk [5] draw on the software design, development and testing literatures that identify there are many blunt sources of errors that are software or hardware (e.g. device) oriented that are specific to the software development lifecycle (SDLC). They added to this work by discussing the possible error introducing aspects of the organization who purchases the software and hardware and the possible sources of error that arise from their customization and implementation in the local organization. Borycki and Kushniruk [5] suggested that the SDLC process, when not executed with an understanding of the healthcare environment and an understanding of how poor execution of the processes, may lead to errors. They also recognized the importance of organizational influences upon technology-induced errors - arising from the customization, poor implementation and deployment, and subsequent operation of systems (this being in keeping with the work of Reason [7] attempting to identify the cause of error as arising from the complexities associated with organizational context). Even so the researchers present a limited view of error - limiting it to the SDLC and the local healthcare organization without considering other organizational blunt causes of error that Reason [7] suggests and the multiple organizational influences upon error rates that Orlikowski's [8] theoretical work begins to shed light on as sources of technology-induced error. We suggest that in order to fully understand the blunt causes of error involving technology (i.e. technology-induced errors) there is a need to consider the multiple organizational influences that are present and emerge as a result of the process.

2. The Framework

In this paper the authors present a new framework for diagnosing technology-induced errors that extends Reason's work [7] to the study and prevention of technology-induced error in healthcare and examines the blunt sources of sharp end error (See figure 1). This framework extends Reason's [7] "Swiss cheese model" of system accidents, where high technology systems are seen as having many defensive layers, each of which may have "holes" through which problems may propagate ultimately leading to error. In this model, it is when the holes "line up" that the opportunity for error arises (i.e. allowing for a "trajectory of accident opportunity"). In our extension of this model to health informatics the causes of error can be located on a continuum from blunt end causes shown on the left hand side of Figure 1 (e.g. related to sources such as differences between policy and legislation between jurisdictions that may not be reflected in healthcare information systems) to sharp end causes (e.g related to errors arising from more local situations and individual human work). Orlinkowski [8] in her research identifies that information systems are initially developed by software companies by visiting a model organization and replicating that institutions processes electronically in the information system that is designed and built. If the model organization has ineffective processes, these processes can become embedded within the system by programmers. In turn, these affect the adopting organization. Moving along the continuum from blunt to sharp end, vendor organizations may also introduce errors by automating ineffectual processes borrowed from the model organization. They may also introduce new categories of error through poor requirements gathering, design, programming and failure to sufficiently test their software. Lastly, the local organization implementing a system may introduce opportunities for errors through the process of customization and adaptation of the system to the local environment (e.g. ineffectually modifying a system to be reflective of local workflow, or selecting a device that will not integrate properly with existing devices or systems). In addition, at the level of the local organization adopting a system, lack of attention to training and support may also lead to other categories of errors at the sharp end (i.e. where the individual user interacts with the system).

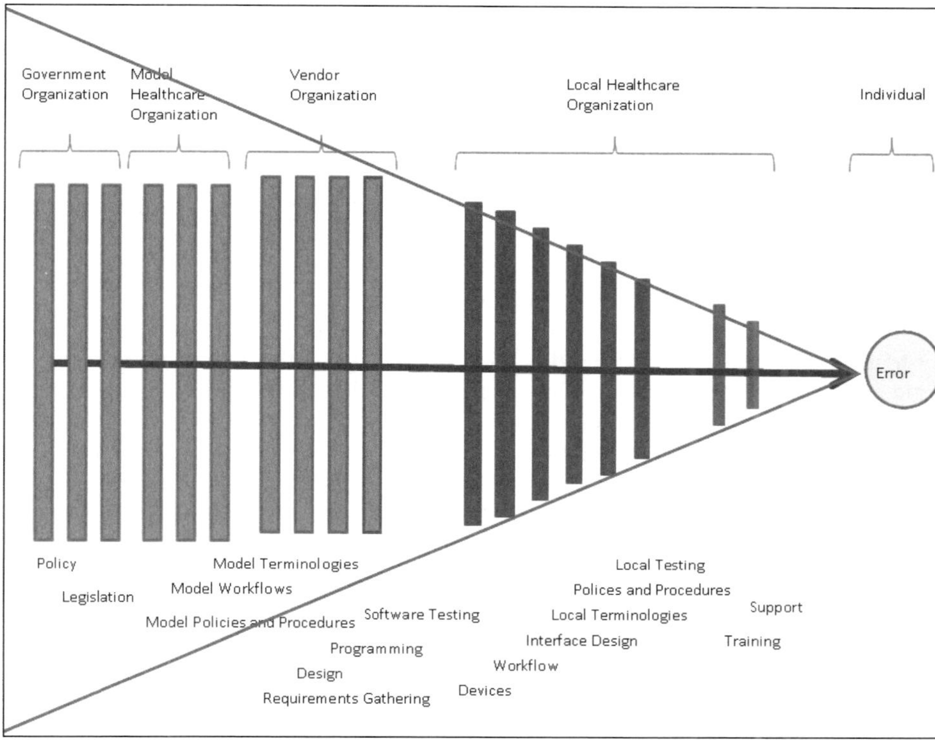

Figure 1: A Framework for Diagnosing Technology-Induced Errors in Healthcare

The authors propose that in order to have a fully robust understanding the of the blunt causes of technology-induced errors one must understand the development of technology and the influences of policy using a multi-organizational framework for diagnosing technology-induced errors. The authors propose that technology-induced errors may have their origins in up to four or more organizations that make up complex health care systems. The first of these structures is the governmental or regulatory organization where health care policy is set and legislation governs the types of technologies that are developed by vendor organizations and are procured and implemented by local healthcare organizations. The second is the model organization that is used to design and develop the software [8]. The third is the vendor who designs, develops, programs and tests the software. The fourth is the local organization that customizes, implements and supports the software and hardware and trains healthcare providers [5].

3. Experiences in Applying the Framework

To date we have used the framework we have described above to guide our research in the study of technology-induced error. For example, we have investigated how system interface features designed by vendors (at the vendor organization level of the model in Figure 1) can ultimately impact error rates in entering prescriptions into a hand-held prescription writing application at the sharp end of the model [3]. In this work we have been able to statistically relate how frequently usability problems embedded by vendors in the system interface are associated with actual medication errors. Some specific user interface problems (e.g. display visibility problems) were found to be highly related to errors made by physicians in entering medications into the prescription writing application (with up to 80% of such identified usability problems being associated with medication error during usability testing). In other related recent work we have extended this research to apply computer based simulations to forecast the impact of specific user interface design features on errors at the sharp end (i.e. medication errors made by health care providers using medication administration systems) [19].

Moving further forward along the continuum in Figure 1 we have also extended the use of the framework to the study of the interaction between a health information system and the devices that are used at point of care. Here, the interaction between the rigid workflows programmed by the vendor and devices selected by an organization were shown to lead to health care provider workarounds (e.g. subjects indicated they would need to skip procedures involving the system and device during emergencies to accomplish a task) [13]. In this series of studies it was found that inability to customize or modify work processes embedded in the vendor product studied was a significant source of technology-induced medication error.

We are currently extending our work to examine the impact of policy and legislation when incorporated into the design and development of systems. For example, privacy laws, when incorporated into system design, may prevent some health care providers from obtaining sufficient information to make a decision. We are also planning to investigate the impact of use of model organizations upon software design and their downstream effects upon the vendor and local organizations through observation of model organizations and how their processes are reflected in the systems design and the adopting organization and their subsequent effects upon the health care providers working in the adopting organization.

4. Conclusions

As we increasingly begin to use health information systems in the day-to-day functioning of health care organizations, researchers need to develop new methods of identifying and addressing technology-induced errors at the blunt end before they emerge as errors at the sharp end involving patients and health care providers. There is a need to develop and test new models of representing technology-induced errors in health care. Health care is considered to be as unique and complex as the nuclear power and airline industries which have developed industry specific methods of evaluating blunt end impacts upon sharp end activities. In the next few years researchers in the health and biomedical informatics domain will need to develop similar methods and frameworks to diagnose the causes of error that are health care specific. Furthermore, there will be a need for researchers to test these models for their ability to diagnose or identify the blunt source of error after an accident has occurred to prevent the error from occurring again. There will also be a need to develop methods and frameworks with predictive abilities to prevent errors from occurring. Addressing technology-induced errors is a difficult process when one considers the multiple complex organizations that may influence an error occurring at the sharp end (i.e. when the holes in the Swiss Cheese model align and an error occurs). Governments and regulatory bodies will need to address the blunt end sources of technology-induced errors as there is a need for an integrated approach to identifying sources of error and no one organization is fully responsible in the current healthcare system. Ultimately, governments, model organizations (used in the design of software), organizations that design software, local health care organizations and the individual all have a role in the errors occurring at the sharp end.

References

[1] Levenson N. Safeware: System safety and computers. Reading, Massachusetts: Addison-Wesley, 2004.
[2] Koppel R, Metlay JP, Cohen A, Abaluck B, Localio AR, Kimmel SE, Strom BL. Role of computerized physician order entry systems in facilitating medication errors. JAMA. 2005; 293(10): 1197-1203.
[3] Kushniruk AW, Triola MM, Borycki EM, Stein B, Kannry JL. Technology induced error and usability: The relationship between usability problems and prescription errors when using a handheld application. Int J Med Inform. 2005; 74(7-8): 519-526.
[4] Ash JS, Sittig DF, Dykstra R, Campbell E, Guappone K.. The unintended consequences of computerized provider order entry: Findings from a mixed methods exploration. Int J Med Inform. 2009; 78(1): S69-76.
[5] Borycki EM, Kushniruk AW. Where do technology-induced errors come from? In AW Kushniruk and EM Borycki (Eds.). Human, social and organizational aspects of health information systems. Hershey, New York: IGI Global: 2008.
[6] Joint Commission for Health Care Quality. Sentinel event alert. 42(1), http://www.jointcommission.org/SentinelEvents/SentinelEventAlert/se_42.htm
[7] Reason J. Human error: Models and management. BMJ. 320: 768-770.
[8] Orlinkowski WJ. The duality of technology: Rethinking the concept of technology in organizations. Organization Science. 1992; 3(3): 398-427.
[9] Vicente K. The human factor: Revolutionizing the way we live with technology. Toronto: Vintage Canada: 2003.
[10] Woods D, Cook RI. The new look at error, safety and failure: A primer for health care. Chicago: National Patient Safety Foundation.
[11] Horsky J, Kuperman GJ, Patel VL. Comprehensive analsysi of a medication dosage related error related to CPOE. JAMIA. 2005; 12 (4): 377-382.
[12] Patel VL, Currie LM. Clinical cognition and biomedical informatics: Issues of patient safety. Int J Med Inform, 74(11-12): 869-885.
[13] Kushniruk AW, Borycki EM, Kuwata S, Watanabe H. Using a low-cost simulation approach for assessing the impact of a medication administration system on workflow. In SK Andersen et al. (Eds.) eHealth beyond the horizon: Get IT there. Amsterdam: IOS Press.
[14] Keay, E., Kushniruk, AW. The development of a risk identification screening framework for healthcare information systems. In J.G. McDaniel (Ed.) Advances in Information Technology and Communications in Health. IOS Press, 2009, 400-405.
[15] Borycki EM, Kushniruk AW, Kuwata S, Watanabe H. Simulations to assess medication administration systems. In B. Staudinger, V. Hoess and H. Osterman (Eds.). Nursing and Clinical Informatics. Hershey, Pennsylvania: IGI.
[16] George M, Rowlands D, Kastle B. What is lean six sigma? Toronto: McGraw Hill.
[17] Kushniruk AW, Borycki EM, Kuwata S, Kannry J. Predicting changes in workflow resulting from healthcare information systems: Ensuring the safety of healthcare. Healthc Q. 2006; 9: 114-118.
[18] Beuscart-Zephir MC, Pelayo S, Anceaux, F, Meaux JJ, Degroisse M, Degoulet P. Impact of CPOE on doctor-nurse cooperation for the medication ordering and administration process. Int J Med Inform. 2005; 74(7-8): 629-641.
[19] Kushniruk AW, Borycki EM, Anderson JG, Anderson MM. Combining two forms of simulation to predict the potential impact of interface design on technology-induced error in healthcare. SpringSim. 2008: 497-504

Detection and Prevention of Adverse Drug Events
R. Beuscart et al. (Eds.)
IOS Press, 2009

doi:10.3233/978-1-60750-043-8-188

Gaming Against Medical Errors: Methods and Results from a Design Game on CPOE

Anne Marie KANSTRUP [a,1], Christian NØHR [b]
[a] *Department of Communication, Aalborg University.*
[b] *Department of Development and Planning, Aalborg University*

Abstract. The paper presents design game as a technique for participatory design for a Computerized Decision Support System (CDSS) for minimizing medical errors. Design game is used as a technique for working with the skills of users, the complexity of the use practice and the negotiation of design here within the challenging domain of medication. The paper presents a developed design game based on game inspiration from a computer game, theoretical inspiration on electronic decision support, and empirical grounding in scenarios of medical errors. The game has been played in a two-hour workshop with six clinicians. The result is presented as a list of central themes for design of CDSS and derived design principles from these themes. These principles are currently under further exploration in follow up prototype based activities.

Keywords. Design game, decision support, medical error

"Understanding people as "actors" in situations, with a set of skills and shared practices based on work experience with others, requires us to seek new ways of understanding the relationship between people, technology, work requirements, and organizational constraints in work settings. Studying such a multi-faceted and multi-layered issue requires that we go beyond more traditional controlled laboratory studies that are the hallmark of experimental human-computer interaction (HCI) studies" [1].

Introduction

In this paper we present the use of design games for engaging clinicians in the design of computerized decision support for minimizing medical errors. As stated in the initial quotation of Bannon [1] our background for working with participation and activities like games is based on participatory design perspectives on

- Users as competent professionals and thus powerful active agents in design of software to support the quality of their own practice
- Practice as complex and thus calling for situated studies to, if not grasp then at least, sense the complexity of real world situations
- Design as negotiation and a social construction process – there is no truth out there, thus, design process with participation of central actors and iterations making space for learning is central.

1 Corresponding Author: kanstrup@hum.aau.dk

These participatory principles for design of computer systems (see e.g. [2] for elaboration) are challenged when entering the domain of medication in hospitals as dealt with in this study: Hospitals are short on resources, i.e. using clinicians' time for design activities always means taking their time away from patient care. Hospital wards are busy and subject to ethical issues towards patients, i.e. entering a hospital ward as researcher or designer of computer systems is always disturbing and problematic. Medical work is evidence based. Thus, explorative and iterative design processes are difficult. In the following we present how we have worked with the technique of design game as a step in a design process for CDSS to minimize medication errors. The design game made it possible to work with our participatory design principles within the domain of medication at hospital wards.

The study presented is part of the European project PSIP (Patient Safety through Intelligent Procedures in medication), which aims to identify and prevent adverse drug events (ADE). The main objective of the project is to develop innovative knowledge based on data mining results and to deliver to professionals and patients a contextualized knowledge fitting the local risk parameters in the form of alerts and decision support functions. The designs of these decision support functions are the aim of the design game approach.

1. Design Games

Games have been used for several years within participatory design [3] and several types of exploratory design games have been developed and used in a variety of participatory design processes: games to conceptualize designing, games for exchanging perspectives for design, games for negotiation of workflow, scenario oriented design games [4]. Design games are interesting and a relevant technique since

- Design games are a framework accommodating the challenging collaboration between people with various competencies and interests [4].
- Design games are a reflective activity. The activity of designing a game to bring out ideas for design is producing the rules for the design process in which it is going to be used and at the same time it is a reflection upon the action of design [3].

Games were introduced in participatory design to provoke the development of a shared understanding among the players, users and designers alike and to form a basis for dialogue [5]. Likewise, the game must help moving beyond an under-standing of the current practice and generate ideas for future design [6, 7]. As pointed out by Kanstrup & Christiansen [3] the workings of the opening of the mind that gaming generates can be explained by Bateson's reflections on fun and seriousness, fantasy and games [8, pp. 14-26 and 177-200). Bateson calls attention to the characteristics of games as a serious business in which we are able to generate new ideas by playing at unknown paths [8, p. 17]. Playing is an exploration of the rules of order, a "muddle" which gets us "somewhere" [8, p. 19). The exploration of the rules for what makes something "for real" and something "for fun" is part of the experimentation of design – but it is also what makes gaming playful.

2. The Incredible Machine as Game Inspiration

The design game for CDSS was made on game inspiration from the computer game "the incredible machine", a theoretical understanding of electronic decision as four levels, and empirical understanding of medication errors translated to a set of scenarios for gaming.

For the game setting we were inspired by a computer game from the 1980's called "the incredible machine". A screenshot from the main screen in the game is shown in figure 1 [9]. In the middle the main playing field where various objects are each prearranged in fixed position for each level in the game. In the column on the right are a number of functionalities that can be drawn into the field with the mouse. The general objective of the game is to create a series of "Heath Robinson devices[2]"; arrange a given collection of objects in a complex fashion so as to perform some simple task, for example "light a candle". Available functionalities or objects range from simple ropes and pulleys to electrical generators, bowling balls, and even monkeys, cats, and mice. In the bottom of the screen the scores are kept.

In the PSIP design game the scenarios e.g. as shown in figure 2 were the main playing field, and the functionalities were either predefined e.g. as shown in figure 3 or just blank sheets of paper where the participants could write their own ideas of a functionality.

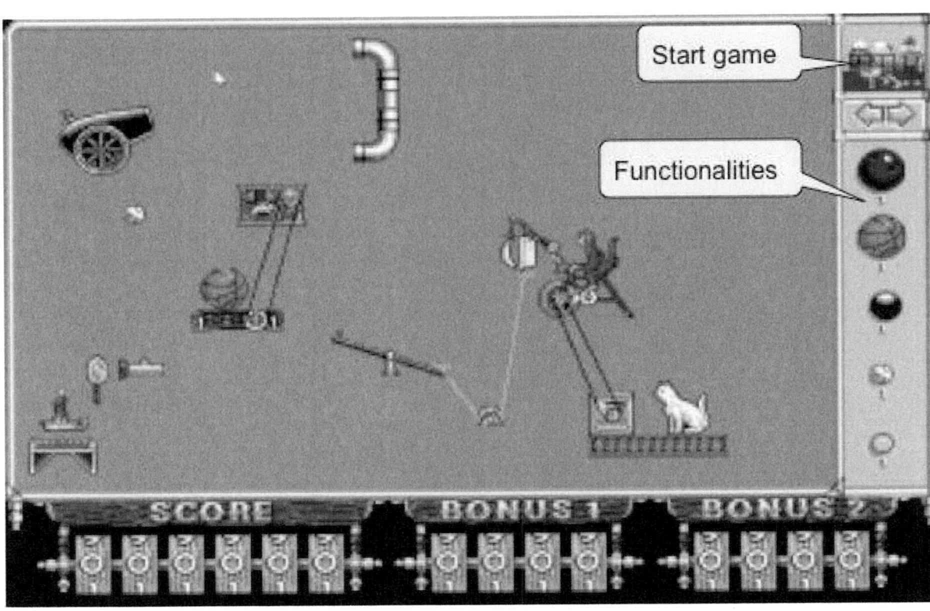

Figure 1. Screenshot from "The Incredible Machine

[2] Heath Robinson was an English cartoonist and illustrator, who is known for drawings of eccentric machines and "Heath Robinson" has entered the language as a description of any unnecessarily complex and implausible contraption.

3. A Theoretical Perspective on Decision Support

The theoretical basis for the core of the game is founded in four identified levels for electronic decision support [10, 11]:

7. Base level of categorized information that requires further processing and analysis by users before a decision could be made.
8. An opportunistic focus of the clinician's attention by prompts, reminders, or alerts about out of range assessment results and intervention strategies.
9. More complex consultation advice based on deductive inference engines, which operate on some knowledge base and automatically generate diagnostic or intervention recommendations.
10. Automated prompts and advices on patient and situation specific issues by means of artificial intelligence techniques including self-learning capabilities and fuzzy set formalisms.

4. Scenarios for Empirical Grounding

To ensure an empirical grounding, i.e. understanding of the complex practice of medication, the game is based on a number of scenarios made from actual cases reported as patient safety incidents. The Cases has been retrieved from the National Danish database for adverse incidents reports. The reported data in the database has been edited to match the generic taxonomy as shown in figure 2.

Incident	
	The patient is admitted for a suspected joint infection. Instead an attack of gout is diagnosed. NSAID is prescribed which betters the attack of gout. Three days later the patient develops epistaxis and the warfarin dose has to be lowered.
Patient characteristics	
Age and sex	55 years, male
Weight and height	97 kg, 175 cm
Medical history	
Medications	Enalapril 20 mg x 1, *antihypertensive* Methformine 500 mg x 3, *antidiabetic* Simvastatin 40 mg x 1, at night, *cholesterol-lowering* Warfarin 7.5/5.0/7.5/5.0/7.5/5.0/5.0 mg x 1, *anticoagulant*
Prior diagnoses	I10.9 Hypertension E10.2 Diabetes, type II E78.0 Hypercholesterolemia I48.9B Atrial fibrillation M10.0 Gout (metabolic arthritis)
Allergies	No allergies
Current situation	
Lab values	INR 2.3 [2.0-3.0] Creatinine 157 micromol/L [60-130 micromol/L]

	Urate 0.721 mmol/L [0.20-0.45 mmol/L]
Working diagnosis and clinical problem	M10.0 Gout (metabolic arthritis)
Department	Department of internal medicine; admitted from home.
Triggers	
	1. Warfarin/NSAID interaction Class effect, i.e. interaction between *all* NSAID's and warfarin 2. Concurrent prescription of enalapril and NSAID in the presence of elevated creatinine in a diabetic patient presents a risk of aggravating the patient's slight renal insufficiency

Figure 2. Scenario 1: Anticoagulant therapy – interaction[3]

It is considered essential to use real scenarios as it eliminates diverting discussion of the realism. To play the game we had a total of 22 scenarios available.

5. Gaming Against Medical Errors

The PSIP design game was to create a space for users to participate with their design ideas for CDSS. For this reason it was important that the game emphasized focused but creative discussions. We worked on supporting the participants with concrete artifact on what it was that they should design:

- a box called "the PSIP machine" was made as a physical artifact that they could point to, hold, discuss the functionality of – their incredible machine
- a set of laminated scenarios for situations with medical errors (cf. Figure 2) for focusing and situating discussions and designs against medical errors
- a number of pre-made functionalities for electronic decision support were printed and laminated corresponding to the four theoretical levels of decision support [11] Examples of the pre-made functionalities are shown in figure 3.

[3] The scenarios are developed by Brian Bjørn, Jonas Egebart, Unit for Patient Safety, Capital Region, Denmark

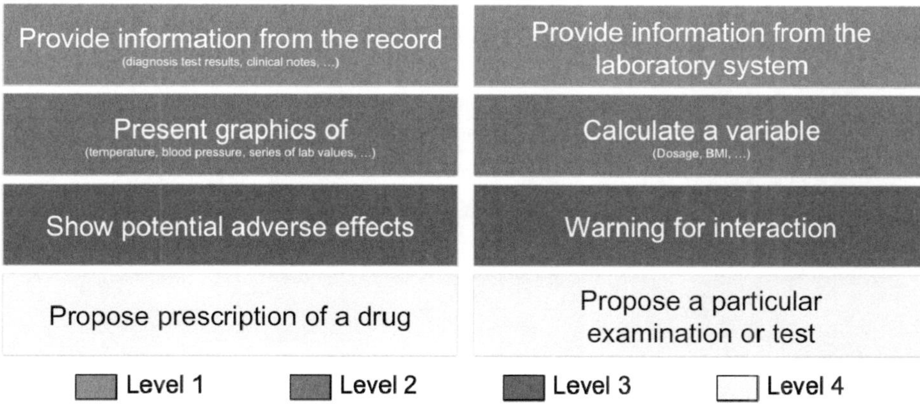

Figure 3. Premade decision support functionalities for design of an incredible decision support machine. The colours correspond to different levels of decision support.

Several actors participated in the game activity:

- A game master explains the rules, facilitates the discussions and keeps the time.
- A point master keeps the scores and facilitates the evaluation of the designed machines.
- Two persons document the process by photos and video.
- Four physicians and two registered nurses are the most important participants in the game

The participants were divided in two competing teams – a green team and a blue team. The task for the teams was to build machines that can help to prevent the errors in the scenarios. There are no limits to the ability of the machines, they can do whatever the participants can imagine – they are incredible.

The schedule of the game is as follows:

- Each individual has two minutes to read the scenario,
- The team has 10 minutes to discuss the scenario and design an incredible decision support machine that can help prevent the adverse drug event in the scenario.
- For design the team can use the pre-developed functionalities or they can make their own functionality on blank paper
- After the 10 minutes of discussion and design the teams were allowed two minutes each to present their solution. The score master considered each solution and points were given to each team. The use of a pre-made functionality was given one point while self-made suggestions gave five points.
- After one hour of designing machines the teams were given a break. During the break the game master displayed the design suggestion on a table and subsequently the teams prioritized and commented each other's machines and ideas.

The game process and the results were documented with video and photos.

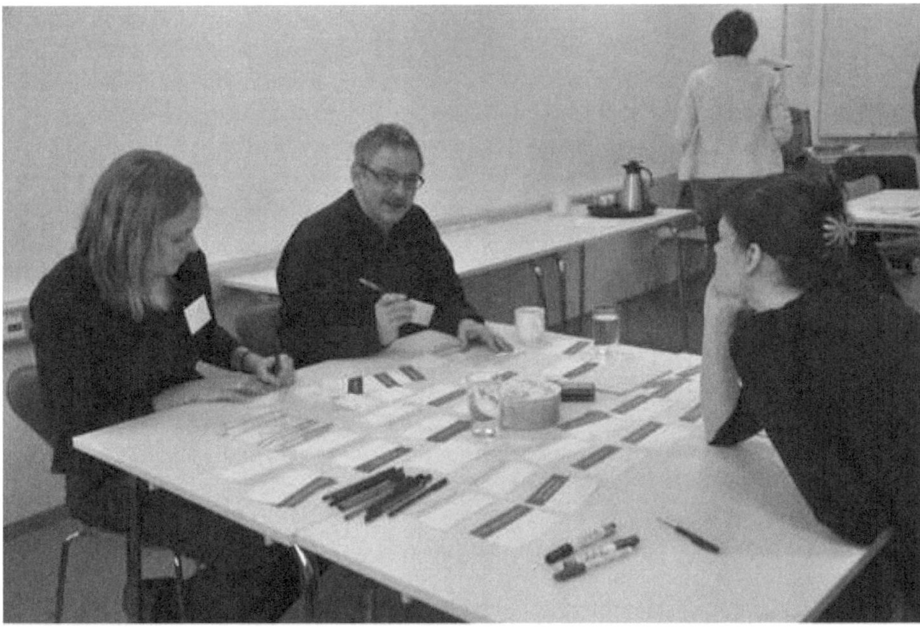

Figure 4. Green team in the design game

6. Game Results

The result of the design game was eight incredible machines for decision support preventing medical errors. These "machines" presented what the participants found as central foci related to medical errors and decision support. Figure 5 lists these themes in an order as prioritized by the players: in the left column central themes from the participants design and in the right column the design principles that the authors have derived for CDSS design.

Theme	Design Principle
Risks related to lack of integration of information	**Design for integrated information:** if physicians are to gather information from several different information systems the risk that some information will be missing is high. Hand written information is dangerous and must be avoided.
	Integrated information must be used intelligently for clinical alerts, i.e. in cases of interaction.
Risks related to misreading and analysis of measurements and test results	**Design graphical diagrams for visualizing measurements and lab results**: diagrams, eg. a curve, will at a glance reveal if a measurement is out of normal range.
Risks related to rigid information	**Design for optimizing prescription:**

systems	Information systems experienced as rigid and a disturbance (vs. a support) of the clinical work tend to lead to bad data discipline and workarounds.
Risks related to interruptions	**Design for calm working environments when prescribing dispensing and administering medicine.**
Risk related to misreading of medicine	**Design for barcode readings** or other types of scanning for verification.

Figure 5. Results (themes and derived principles) from the player's designs.

7. Discussion

The result of the design game is not a list of features to implement but a list of themes related to risk of errors identified by skilled actors in work practices. Returning to the initial Bannon quote these themes bring us closer to an understanding of the relationship between people, technology, work requirements and organizational constraints in work settings [1]. The list highlights not only requirements for interfaces between systems but also problems of interruptions, misreading in a high tempo work environment, and shortcuts made when systems are experienced as barriers and not supporters of work practices.

From a resource perspective the two-hour design game provided central knowledge and ideas for future design. From a design perspective the game technique provided negotiations between skilled users on complex practices and ideas for solutions.

Design concepts based on these design principles are in progress and mock-ups of design concepts will be exposed to critical discussion with the players of the game in a workshop and subsequently, design concepts will be implemented to a running prototype for exploration in a scenario based evaluation.

8. Conclusion

The paper has presented design game as a technique for participatory design for CDSS. A design game has been presented based on game inspiration from the computer game "the incredible machine", theoretical inspiration on electronic decision support as four levels, and empirical grounding in scenarios of medical errors. The game has been played in a two-hour workshop with six clinicians. The design game resulted in eight incredible designs, user discussions and priorities of designs and from this a list of central themes that the players pointed out for design of CDSS and derived design principles from these themes.

In short, the design game provided central knowledge and ideas for future design based on negotiations from skilled users on complex practices and ideas for solutions. Further research will develop concepts and design prototypes on this basis and explore these in follow up participatory activities.

Acknowledgements

The research leading to these results has received funding from the European Community's Seventh Framework Programme (FP7/2007-2013) under grant agreement n°216130 – The PSIP project. Thanks to the participating clinicians from hospitals in the Capital Region in Copenhagen, and to the colleagues from the PSIP project.

References

[1] Bannon, Liam: "From Human Factors to Human Actors: The Role of Psychology and Human-Computer Interaction Studies in Systems Design" in Joan Greenbaum & Morten Kyng (eds.): Design at Work: cooperative design of computer systems. Lawrence Erlbaum Associates. Hillsdale, New Jersey, 1991.
[2] Greenbaum, J. & Kyng, M. Design at Work, Lawrence Erlbaum ass. 1991
[3] Kanstrup, A. M. & Christiansen, E. "Designing Games – balancing fun and seriousness" in Proceedings of the Danish HCI Research Symposium DHRS 2005. Copenhagen Business School.
[4] Brandt, E. Designing exploratory design games: a framework for participation in Participatory Design? In Proceedings of the ninth conference on Participatory design: Expanding boundaries in design – volume 1. August 2006, Trento, Italy.
[5] Ehn, P. & Sjøgren, D.: From systems Descriptions to Scripts for Action in: Greenbaum, J. & Kyng, M. Design at Work, Lawrence Erlbaum ass. 1991
[6] Johansson, M. & Linde, P. "Playful Collaborative Exploration: New Research Practice in Participatory Design". In Journal of Research Practice, Vol. 1, Issue 1, Article M5, 2005.
[7] Bødker, S. & Christiansen, E. "Scenarios as springboards in design" in Bowker, G., Gaser, L., Star, S.L. & Turner, W. (Eds.) Social Science research, technical systems and cooperative work, Erlbaum, Mahwah, NJ, 217-234.
[8] Bateson, G. Steps to an Ecology of Mind. The University of Chicago Press, Chicago, 2000 (1972).
[9] Wikipedia: http://en.wikipedia.org/wiki/The_Incredible_Machine Accesses 20. April 2009
[10] Liaw S T, Schattner P: Electronic decision support in general practice. What's the hold up?, Australian Family Physician Vol. 32, no. 11, November 2003. P. 941-944
[11] NICT: Report of the electronic decision support governance workshop. Melbourne: National Institute of Clinical Studies, November 2001.

Detection and Prevention of Adverse Drug Events
R. Beuscart et al. (Eds.)
IOS Press, 2009

doi:10.3233/978-1-60750-043-8-197

The PSIP Approach to Account for Human Factors in Adverse Drug Events: Preliminary Field Studies

Costanza RICCIOLI[a,1], Nicolas LEROY[b] and Sylvia PELAYO[b]
[a] *KITE Solutions, SNC, Via Labiena 93, 21014 Laveno Mombello (Va), Italy*
[b] *Evalab, CIC-IT Lille, University Hospital of Lille, France*

Abstract. This paper presents a preliminary contribution of a Human Factors (HF) approach to prevention of Adverse Drug Events (ADEs), developed within the European research project Patient Safety through Intelligent Procedures in medication (PSIP). Following an introduction on the role and relevance of HF in ADEs prevention, a number of systemic weaknesses encountered during the field activity analysis are presented and discussed. Semi-structured interviews and observations of medication cycle activities led to infer potential unreliability of some decision-making and drug administration procedures. In particular, the usage of current electronic support systems emerged as a crucial related element. These findings represent an initial contribution which will be further developed within PSIP, as HF have been recognised fundamental contributors to ADEs epidemiological knowledge and appropriate prevention.

Keywords. Adverse Drug Event, Human Factors, systemic approach, ethnographic study, Computerised Decision Support System

Introduction

Adverse Drug Events (ADEs) have been defined as injuries related to the use, administration or prescribing of a drug [1,2,3]. Preventable ADEs are accounted as any unwanted consequence caused by the use or non-use of a drug due to errors that can occur at various stages of the medication cycle.

ADEs prevention focuses on two main areas: (1) the understanding of the general causes at the base of individual errors and of the amplification of their consequences; and (2) the electronic supporting of work activities that are cognitively complex, as decision-making (diagnosis and prescription), or easily prone to confusion, as drug preparation and (auto)administration, e.g., wrong patient, drug, dose, etc.

The two approaches are not mutually exclusive; on the contrary they are frequently merged [4] with excellent results.

The recognised major cause of preventable ADEs is "human error" [5]. Therefore, the usual measures of safety of patient, namely, prevention or recovery from situations at risk when errors have not been prevented, and containment of the consequences, if prevention and recovery have not been successful, have been developed and implemented.

[1] Corresponding Author: costanza.riccioli@kitesolutions.it

As an example, there is a growing diffusion in hospitals of different kinds of electronic systems supporting several medical activities and management [6], as *Computer Physician Order Entry* (CPOE), that support in particular the sharing of treating instruction and patient medical history, and *Clinical Decision Support Systems* (CDSS) for decision-makers.

These systems help substantially in reducing the contribution of "human error" to the number of ADEs, at prevention and containment of the consequences. However, a more in-depth assessment of the root causes of errors has to be tackled, so as to identify and eliminate the "pathological" roots of human errors.

The Human Factors (HF) research on errors focuses nowadays on the analysis and detection of the organizational and systemic causes that lead to individual mistakes. The focus is not only on human cognitive or social characteristics, as in psychological studies, but on the *interaction* between them and the elements of the working context, including tools and technologies [7]. Methods as the *Root cause analysis* are able to account for active (visible) errors occurred, as well as for latent conditions that favour and contribute in creating error manifestations [8].

This paper presents the general theoretical framework on human errors that sustains a field study conducted within the European research project PSIP, which aims to take into account both the ADEs prevention areas, designing a Human Factors oriented support system to medication cycle activities and individual actors[2].

1. The PSIP Project

The European project *Patient Safety through Intelligent Procedures in medication* (PSIP) has started at the beginning of 2008 with the aim to reduce ADEs number and consequences by achieving two main sub-objectives.

The first one is to facilitate the systematic production of epidemiological knowledge on ADEs, namely, their number, type, consequences and causes, including Human Factors. A list of observed ADEs, with associated frequencies and probabilities, has been created from data mining of hospitals databases and semantic mining of free-texts (letters, reports).

The second sub-objective is to ameliorate the entire medication cycle in a hospital environment by ADEs prevention. The innovative knowledge based on the mining results, after fitting a number of "contextualised" local parameters, is currently being implemented in a new platform, in the form of alerts and decision support functions. Existing ICT (Information and Communication Technologies) applications can connect to the platform to access and integrate the knowledge in their local system.

Data mining is the process of automatically searching large volumes of data for patterns using different tools, such as decision trees, association rules, Logistic Regression Analysis, Multi-factorial Analysis, etc. Semantic mining identifies patterns and trends from texts by means of statistical pattern learning. The main advantage of those techniques is the possibility to quickly analyse extensive numbers of data related to real patients and stays, including occurred injuries due or related to ADEs.

In the PSIP project, mining processes have extracted the most frequently encountered associations between patient diseases, characteristics, drugs and negative

[2] The research leading to these results has received funding from the European Community's Seventh Framework Program (FP7/2007-2013) under grant agreement n° 216130.

outcomes that represent a very valuable contribution in terms of ADEs epidemiological knowledge. However, HF contributions to ADEs, which are fundamental for prevention or mitigation of consequences, are difficult to obtain by means of such methods, as current medical databases and texts are very poor in information on possible ADEs human related basic causes.

The implementation of HF methods research is therefore an essential parallel component of the project. This process takes place in three steps: first of all, the results deriving from mining techniques are verified by human experts to assure their ecological validity. Secondly, the existing mining results can be enriched with field studies to identify error causes and contextualise them. Thirdly, the new support platform is being designed with a user-centred approach and with the contribution of HF findings.

2. The Analysis of Two Wards Activity: A Field Study

2.1. Rationale of the Study

The assessment of HF contribution to ADEs that embraces the whole medical working and technological environments, and not only the human beings actively involved in the events, is usually referred as “systemic approach”. The need to perform a series of field studies in this perspective, has been recognised essential within the context of the PSIP project for several reasons.

A first one is the possibility to integrate data and semantic mining detection of errors with a systemic analysis of human error: the identification of the errors and the weaknesses of a system by analysing its work organization and individuals [9]. According to this approach individual errors turn into serious consequences (those that mining techniques take into account) only if the entire *system* allows it. This means that the focus for early detection and prevention should shift from individual errors to organizational weaknesses, the so-called *latent factors* [8].

Secondly, the study of real contexts is important so as to integrate innovative instruments, as the final PSIP platform, within real work activities. The “Usability Engineering” and “Contextualisation of CDSS Modules” of the project will design the new support system in a user-centred way. This enables also the development of adaptive interfaces to different kinds of users (physicians, pharmacists, nurses, patients) within different activities (diagnosis, validation, dispensation, administration, self-medication) in different local contexts. Local activity analysis is therefore an important and essential element of this process.

The present study aims at the initial collection of field data in one of the hospitals involved in the mining collection of ADEs.

2.2. Study Site

The Centre Hospitalier de Denain is a 621-bed General Hospital located in the North of France. It employs 600 people, treating approximately 23000 patients every year.

It was chosen as set of this field study owing to its links to PSIP project themes: (1) the hospital is a source of one of the medical databases analysed with mining techniques; and (2) in the year 2000, following a new Quality Policy, a Hospital

Information System, integrating a Computerised Provider Order Entry (CPOE) System, has been installed in all departments.

In particular, the study involved two wards: *Médecine A* (Gastroenterology - Cardiology) and *Médecine B* (Internal Medicine - Infectious Diseases).

2.3. Methodology

An activity analysis has been performed using some standard Human Factors methods of the so-called *ethnographic studies* [10,11,12]: interviews (semi-structured) and observations.

We interviewed two nurses per ward. The interview structure consisted in a list of questions concerning a typical day of work: activities, times, procedures, tools.

Interviews lasted 30 minutes on average and were digitally audio recorded and transcribed for the analysis.

Different sessions of observations were also conducted in both wards.

In *Médecine A* (*MA*) ward we observed:

- a Cardiology medical round;
- a Cardiology nurses handover;
- a Gastroenterology medical round;
- preparation of medications.

In *Médecine B* (*MB*) ward:

- a nurses, physicians and interns briefing;
- medical round of the first part of the ward;
- medical round of the second part of the ward;
- preparation of medications.

Written notes and some digital photos were taken during the sessions. Due to PSIP research themes, we focused in particular on medications prescription and administration and on the use of electronic support systems, even if we tried not to miss out any element useful to understand the general activities.

In order to minimize the so-called Hawthorne effect[13] excessive spatial and spoken interference with nurses and physicians were avoided.

2.4. Results

The wards activity is described following the widely used Software-Hardware-Environment-Liveware model (SHELL) [14]. Originally developed for the aviation domain, this model enables not only the description of the four basic components of a working domain, but it focuses in particular on their *interactions* with humans (*Liveware*), which is the crucial component in a HF systemic perspective. This central element is affected by the existing *Software*, i.e., rules, habits, practices regulations, norms, and procedures (L-S interaction). It utilises *Hardware*, i.e., physical sources, such as equipment, materials, interfaces, and machines (L-H interaction). It cooperates and interacts with other human beings (L-L interaction). Finally, it is indirectly influenced by *Environment*, which consists in physical, economic, political and social factors (L-E interaction).

The following description of the components interactions within the two wards includes only the elements directly observed or derived from the interviews. Therefore, L-S concerns the actual human procedures and practices in medical rounds, briefings, handovers and preparation of medications. L-H is relative to the interaction with the supports, both formal and informal. In this study, as we observed only the physical environment, the L-E description accounts only for that type of interaction and not for the economic, political and social influences usually included in the L-E analysis.

2.4.1. Liveware-Software

Medical rounds represent one of the central activities of wards.

Both *MA* et *MB* are divided in two sections, and there are two medical rounds every day per ward. In *MA*, each observed round was conducted by a physician and a nurse. It was quite fast, with the nurse displaying and updating the therapy on the laptop, and the physician examining the patient and the results of exams before deciding the therapy and dictating it to the nurse.

On the contrary, in *MB*, medical rounds were performed by interns (alone, or two by two, or with a physician). They entered the patient room only for the medical examination, but they discussed results and changes on the therapy in the corridor.

We observed another fundamental activity with regards to ADEs: the **preparation of medications**. The procedure was the same in the two wards, but in *MB*, following to a current experimentation, it is committed to two pharmacist's assistants, whereas in *MA* it is done by a standard nurse. Medications are prepared in the treatment room, putting administration doses in pill dispensers, one for each patient. The pill dispensers are subdivided in four compartments that correspond to the administration times.

Finally, we observed two **transmissions of information**. They both took place in the nursing rooms. In *MA* it was a nurses handover following the round. All the available nurses were present, not only the two directly involved. The morning shift nurse dictated important information and changes to the following shift nurse. In *MB*, we observed a briefing preceding the round. The transmission was more like a discussion, a collective reasoning involving the intern, the physician and two nurses.

2.4.2. Liveware-Hardware

The hospital is equipped with a complete Patient Care Information System (PCIS) including the MEDASYS DxCare® component. It combines the functions of a CPOE and a patient record, and it is interfaced with the DxPharm® pharmacy system. CPOE functions are available for laboratory, radiology and medication orders and for nurses orders.

It is installed on a certain number of laptops on trolleys, and on the computers of the nursing rooms.

We noticed some remarkable differences concerning its use:

- during the medical round: in *MA* it was used especially by nurses, inside the patient room, to display information and results and to enter new data. One physician out of two had his own additional laptop. In *MB*, the software was used for the same tasks, but by interns and physicians (one laptop for all), and outside the room, in the corridor;
- during the transmission of information: it was used as support in both wards, but in *MA* handover nurses utilized almost only their own sheet, while in *MB*

interns, physicians and nurses based their discussion more on the software and on paper results and documents;
- regarding the preparation of medications: in *MA* the nurse based the whole activity on the software; in *MB* the pharmacist's assistants used only paper documents.

The **nurse personal sheet** is the second remarkable support that was observed. They are informal supporting tools that nurses use to note down the most important changes and information to be communicated during the handover. Its fundamental role was remarked during the interviews. In *MB* the interns had similar sheets too.

2.4.3. Liveware Environment

In each ward the patient rooms are organised in two sections.

Both wards moreover present:
- a nursing room: it is a large room equipped with computers, whiteboards, a medication wall, trolleys, etc. It is the centre of the staff activity.
- a staff room: where nurses and physicians take coffee-breaks and some handovers;
- the head nurse office. In *MA* laptops were here for recharge.
- doctors office.

2.4.4. Liveware-Liveware

We observed **standard** cooperation and/or exchanges between
- physicians - nurses (medical rounds in *MA*, briefing in *MB*);
- physicians - physicians (rounds and briefing in *MB*);
- physicians and nurses - patients (medical rounds);
- nurses - nurses (handover in *MA*);
- pharmacist's assistant - pharmacist's assistant (preparation of medication in *MB*).

We noticed also **non-standard** exchanges, for example patients spontaneously giving important information on their surgical history during the exam; nurses that accidentally pointed out a potential drug adverse effect to interns who were doing the round; a physician who called a colleague from another ward for a qualified advice.

2.5. Discussion

We observed several activities related to the medication cycle showed in Figure 1.

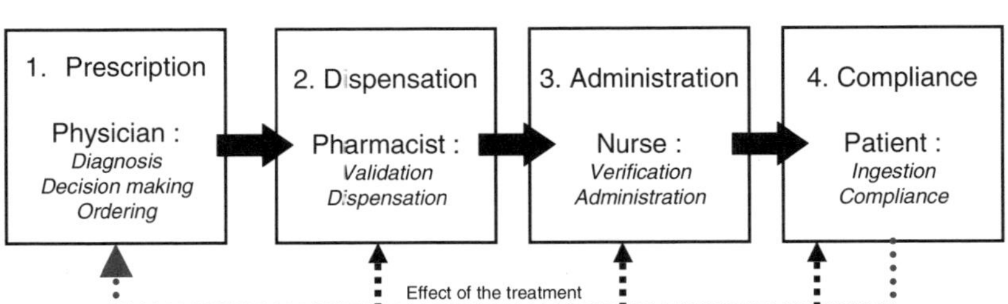

Figure 1. The medication cycle

Medical rounds and briefings are the fundamental circumstances for physicians to gather information useful for the diagnosis and decision-making on therapy; the preparation of medications is part of nurses drugs administration.

Decision-making is a complex cognitive activity. Physicians have to take into account various information from different sources, selecting the most important ones to avoid prescription errors or diagnosis mistakes[15] Our analysis showed a typical distributed management of information between physicians, nurses, patients, paper supports and the software Dx-Care®. This distribution is useful both to lower physician cognitive load and to prevent errors from a systemic point of view. The different information sources and management are all potential defences ("barriers") to accidents pathway [8]. In particular, Dx-Care® contains all the useful information.

However, during our observations, sometimes the information gathering process seemed mostly addressed to individual attention and insights rather than to the software recorded data. Indeed, several differences emerged between the two wards. The medical round in *MA* was faster, conducted by a single decision-maker and a nurse, and the Dx-Care® seemed less taken into account by the physicians, given that there were nurses to display and enter data. In *MB*, two decision-makers took a slower round with a single laptop more largely consulted. As the extensive consultation of Dx-Care® is time consuming, we can infer that the different duration is due to a different usage of the software in the two wards, depending on different actors involved and procedures.

The introduction of a decision support, as the PSIP platform, seems advisable, because it would help in managing multiple information, possibly by giving prominence and alerts to the most serious potential errors causes, and would promote and engender an extensive consultation, which remains a valuable defence against errors.

The second observed activity, the preparation of the medications (part of drug "Administration" in figure 1), even if less related to reasoning, is open to potential important information losses or distractions. These can lead to select the wrong patient, drug or dose. In one case (*MA*), the activity of a single nurse aided by Dx-Care® was observed; in the second ward (*MB*), the activity was conducted by two specialized pharmacist's assistants, using paper documents. These situations are characterized with different defenses to error. In particular, in *MA* the nurse is part of the ward staff, so she is most aware of ward patients and diseases. The activity is driven by the software that can be of support also for cross checks in case of doubts. In *MB*, the pharmacist's assistants are different actors than standard nurses: they are responsible only of drugs dispensing and preparation. Being two, they can easily support each other preventing confusions even if they use paper documents only. In *MA*, the redundancy (a barrier to error) is represented by the software aid. In *MB*, the pharmacist's assistants, even though more qualified about the medications and working as a team, have a minor knowledge of the ward; in fact, a hazard of potential patient confusion due to a homonymy was observed. This represents a potential systemic weakness, joint to the fact that their activity is not supported by Dx-Care®.

In this work "Dispensation" and "Compliance" stages of the medication cycle showed in figure 1 have been not observed; further studies within the PSIP project will apply the HF approach to these activities.

3. Conclusions

In this paper, the initial activity analysis of two wards, conducted within the framework of the European project PSIP, has been presented. Following a Human Factors research methodology some medication cycle activities have been assessed for potential sources of human errors and mishaps.

In light of the initial findings that have been presented, this work underlines the importance of Human Factors research in PSIP within two main areas of interest, namely: causes of ADEs and contextualization of a support system. In the PSIP project, ADEs have been currently identified only by mining techniques, that do not have access to human related root causes. This study represents a first step towards the ADEs causes detection process. Some potential systemic weaknesses emerged within the two wards observed during the field study. First of all, the Dx-Care® CPOE is a comprehensive source and management of information. However, it seemed not always effectively consulted, probably because of time constraints. This means that shorter procedures are followed, as the use of the sole support sheets during handovers, or the fortuitous acquisition of crucial information. The defence represented by the software is therefore replaced by less reliable individual capabilities.

Although this study is mainly related to the first area of interest, it provides also some basic indications on the relevance of contextualisation of the future PSIP platform within real world activities. In particular, it was found that in medical rounds and handover the primary need of exhaustiveness and selection of crucial information is not always guaranteed. A decision-support system can be therefore appropriate in such activities to avoid drug related errors. A more selective process of identification and prominence of important information would also represent a valuable error defence in preparation of medications.

These initial findings, though rather general and preliminary, are interesting examples of the application of Human Factors methods within the PSIP project. It is advisable that further studies will extend those initial results, in detailing the system analysis within its components, and in finding causal links between systemic weaknesses and the occurring of the ADEs detected through mining techniques. This will help in designing a PSIP support platform really effective within real contexts.

Acknowledgments

The research leading to these results has received funding from the European Community's Seventh Framework Programme (FP7/2007-2013) under grant agreement n° 216130 – the PSIP project.

The authors are grateful to Marie-Catherine Beuscart-Zéphir and Pietro Carlo Cacciabue for their support and help in the performing of field study and data analyses.

References

[1] S. Brown, K. Black, S. Mrochek, A. Wood, et al, RADARx: Recognizing, assessing, and documenting adverse Rx events, Proceedings of the AMIA Annual Symposium (2000), 101–105.
[2] D. C. Classen, S. L. Pestotnik, R. S. Evans, and J. P. Burke, Computerized surveillance of adverse drug events in hospital patients, The Journal Of the American Medical Association 266 (1991), 2847–2851.
[3] R. A. Raschke, B. Gollihare, T. A. Wunderlich, J. R. Guidry, et al, A computer alert system to prevent injury from adverse drug events: Development and evaluation in a community teaching hospital, The Journal Of the American Medical Association 280 (1998), 1317–1320.
[4] C. Safran, D. Rind, B. Bush, P. Jones, K. N. Cytryn, and V. L. Patel, Electronic communication and collaboration in a health care practice, Artificial Intelligence in Medicine 12(2) (1998), 139-153.
[5] L. T. Kohn, J. M. Corrigan, and M. S. Donaldson, To Err is Human: Building a Safer Health System, National Academy Press, Washington, DC, 2000.
[6] D. W. Bates, Using information technology to reduce rates of medication errors in hospitals, British Medical Journal 320(7237) (2000), 788–791.
[7] E. Edwards, Introductory overview. In E. L. Wiener, and D. C. Nagel (Eds.), Human Factors in Aviation, Academic Press, San Diego, CA, 1988.
[8] J. T. Reason, Managing the risks of organizational accidents, Aldershot, Ashgate, 1997.
[9] P. C. Cacciabue and G. Vella, Human factors engineering in healthcare systems: The problem of human error and accident management, International Journal of Medical Informatics, In Press, Corrected Proof, Available online 19 December 2008.
[10] M. H. Agar, The professional stranger: An informal introduction to ethnography, Academic Press, London, 1980.
[11] M. J. Perry, R. Fruchter, and D. Rosenberg, Co-ordinating distributed knowledge: A study into the use of an organisational memory, Cognition Technology and Work 1(3) (1999), 142-152.
[12] A. N. Healey, S. Olsen, R. Davis, and C. A. Vincent, A method for measuring work interference in surgical teams, Cognition Technology and Work 10(4) (2008), 305-312.
[13] S. R. G. Jones, Was there a Hawthorne effect?, American Journal of Sociology 98 (1992), 451-468.
[14] F. H. Hawkins, Human Factors in Flight, Gower, Aldershot, UK, 1987.
[15] M. Hunink, P. Glasziou, J. Siegel, J. Weeks, J. Pliskin, A. Elstein, et al., Decision Making in Health and Medicine: Integrating Evidence and Values, Cambridge University Press, New York, 2001.

Detection and Prevention of Adverse Drug Events
R. Beuscart et al. (Eds.)
IOS Press, 2009

doi:10.3233/978-1-60750-043-8-206

The Problem of Defensive Medicine: Two Italian Surveys

Maurizio CATINO [a, 1] and Simona CELOTTI [b]
[a] *University of Milan – Bicocca (Italy)*
[b] *MD – Az.Osp. San Gerardo Monza (Italy).*

Abstract. Defensive medicine takes place when healthcare personnel modify their behaviour with the aim of reducing their exposure to legal challenges from patients. The phenomenon is directly related to the significant growth in medical malpractice litigation over recent years. This article presents the results of two research surveys aimed at measuring the extent of defensive behaviours on the part of doctors in Italy and at understanding the reasons for them. The first study (the National Study (NS) was conducted in respect of a nation-wide sample of general practitioners, while the second (the Local Study (LS) was conducted in respect of two groups of specialists (surgeons and anaesthetists) in a regional hospital. 77.9% of the general practitioners interviewed for the NS (responses were received from 37% of the 1000 GPs to whom the questionnaire was sent) declared that they had practiced at least one form of defensive medicine during the previous working month. The figure for the LS was 83.3%. This article discusses the factors, such as the blame culture and the increase in medical malpractice litigation, that may lead to defensive behaviours and result in negative effects both in terms of costs and patient safety. A clear need emerges for a different approach to the problem of medical error –at a cultural, organizational and legal level–, just as in the case of other organizations subject to high risk. The deterrent of punishment does not increase the reliability of such organizations, nor does it improve the level of safety in them.

Keywords. Defensive medicine – Blame culture – Human error – Organizational learning – Patient safety.

Introduction

There is broad agreement in the academic literature on the definition of defensive medicine: defensive medicine takes place when healthcare personnel effect unnecessary treatments, or avoid high-risk procedures, with the principle - though not exclusive – aim of reducing their exposure to malpractice litigation. Doctors in particular may prescribe tests, procedures or specialist visits (positive defensive medicine), or, alternatively, avoid high-risk patients or procedures (negative defensive medicine). Defensive medicine constitutes a highly damaging effect of the rise in medical litigation, increasing the cost of healthcare and exposing patients to unnecessary risks. The number of negligence claims against doctors is increasing continuously (by 65% over 10 years in Italy; ANIA, 2007[2]) and the large number of legal initiatives taken by patients have induced many doctors to set in place a defensive

1 Corresponding Authors: maurizio.catino@unimib.it
2 The National Association of Insurance Companies.

"strategy" so as to avoid jeopardizing their careers. The threat of medical malpractice litigation constitutes a major obstacle to improving the reliability of healthcare organizations and patient safety.

This article presents the findings of two Italian research surveys conducted in relation to the issue of defensive medicine. In addition, it seeks to clarify the concept of "blame culture" i.e. that shared mindset wherein, when an accident takes place in an organisation, there is a tendency to try immediately to identify the individuals that gave rise to it, to whom the blame is then attributed. Within this perspective the solutions advanced are primarily of a disciplinary and punitive type, while the organisational context is overlooked. A legal and cultural context oriented exclusively towards the identification of individual responsibilities constitutes one of the major causes of defensive behaviours on the part of doctors. It inhibits healthcare organisations from learning about themselves, thereby running the risk of undermining the quality of the healthcare services provided and increasing their cost.

1. Medical Error and Defense Medicine

1.1. Medical Error: Consequences and Costs

The concept of defensive medicine is closely related to that of medical error. In a healthcare context in which there is a perception on the part of the population as a whole that it is exposed to a high risk of medical error, the possibility arises that this concern will influence the relationship between doctors and patients. A recent European-wide study [1] reported that in Italy 97% of citizens consider the issue of medical error an important health issue. While a similar level of concern was found in a number of other countries (Poland, Lithuania and England), the figure for Italy was much higher than those for France, Germany and Belgium (all below the European average). This situation raises the possibility that patients, considering themselves to have been damaged in the course of healthcare provision, initiate legal action against doctors and that, as a direct consequence, doctors, concerned about the threat to their career posed by such litigation, enact strategies of defensive medicine.

On an international level interest in the study of medical error and patient safety gained momentum throughout the 1990s, culminating in the Institute of Medicine's report *To Err is Human* [2]. In a detailed analysis of a number of studies, this report denounced the phenomenon of malpractice and the preventable deaths stemming from it in American hospitals. Making use of two previous studies conducted in three states (Colorado, Utah and New York), the commission responsible for the report pointed out how for every 100 patients subject to hospitalisation a subset ranging from 2.9 to 3.7% encountered some form of malfunctioning, which in some cases lead to death. It found that 53% of such accidents could have been avoided. Projected onto a national figure of 33.6 million hospitalisations per annum, these figures suggested that between 44,000 and 98,000 patients per annum died as a result of some form of accident. According to this research, then, medical error constitutes the eighth most significant cause of death in the United States, resulting in an economic loss of about 29 billion dollars per year. In the wake of the American report a number of other studies were conducted in various countries in the Western world. These confirmed what had been discovered in relation to the risks involved in medical error and in some cases suggested that they had been underestimated.

Table 1. Summary of results of the international research (Vincent, 2005) [3]

Study	Date of admissions	Number of hospital admissions	Adverse event rate (% admissions)
California Insurance Study	1974	20864	4.65
Harvard Medical Practice Study	1984	30195	3.7
Utah-Colorado	1992	14052	2.9
Australia	1992	14179	16.6
Denmark	1998	1097	9.0
New Zealand	1998	6579	11.2
United Kingdom	1999	1014	10.8
Canada	2000	3745	7.5

A recent study [4] conducted on 74,485 patients in various countries (the United States, Australia, England, New Zealand and Canada) demonstrated that 9.2% of hospitalised patients incur iatrogenous damages, of which 43% are preventable and over half (56.3%) without serious consequences. The effects of medical error are not limited just to the damages incurred by patients and the judicial convictions of healthcare personnel but also extend to the impact that the management of risks and the related compensation payments have on the running of the hospital and its costs. It has been estimated that medical liability premiums in the United States have reached an astounding $26 billion annually, representing a 2,000% increase since 1975 [5]. A similar situation is developing in Italy with an attempt on the part of some insurance companies to move out of the market on account of the “risks” and the excessively high costs. It has been estimated that by 2004 medical liability payments in Italy had reached 413 million Euros per annum. From 1995 to 2005 the number of accident claims rose from a little over 17,000 to about 28,500, constituting an increase of 65% [6]. In particular, accident claims in respect of the insurance policies of individual doctors underwent an even more substantial increase, rising from 5,789 in 1995 to 12,374 in 2005 (+134%), while accident claims in respect of the policies of healthcare institutions rose from 11,444 to 16,085, representing an increase of 41%. As a result, the insurance premiums received prior to the emergence of these trends (2007) proved insufficient to cover the damages awarded and this has lead to an even further increase in the premiums and therefore hospital costs in general.

Malpractice litigation has significant repercussions for doctors in professional, moral and psychological terms, further inducing them to practice defensive medicine. The economic repercussions are particularly significant. The various studies show that many doctors believe that being the object of litigation damages their professional reputation and reduces the demand for their services. Moreover, they state that the litigation process itself results in substantial economic damage in the sense that all the tasks deriving out of the need to deal with judicial procedures involve a considerable loss of time and therefore productivity. Further economic damage derives from the need to take out insurance. Many doctors take out insurance policies on an individual basis and even those covered by hospital insurance policies often feel the need to take out additional cover. The psychological repercussions of litigation, in particular, the loss of self-esteem, are also of considerable importance. The state of anxiety provoked by the need to appear in court, for instance, endures long after the conclusion of the actual case [7,8,9,10,11]. The patient comes to be perceived as a potential antagonist and the caring relationship is compromised by an attitude of excessive prudence [12,13].

1.2. The Blame Culture

When an accident takes place there is a tendency to immediately seek to identify the individual players that have supposedly caused it and to attribute guilt exclusively to them. Within this approach the proposed solutions are mainly disciplinary and the organisational context is overlooked. This Individual Blame Logic (IBL) is an accusatory type of approach which seeks to identify guilty individuals [14]. It is particularly characteristic of criminal law, but is also prevalent in organisations based on a punitive culture [15]. More generally, this approach responds to the wish of society to identify a clear cause for accidents [16]. The underlying assumption of IBL is that people make mistakes because they do not pay enough attention to the tasks they are doing. Thus, it adopts a linear causal model, leaving the organisational context for the most part in the background. As a consequence, efforts to identify blame are directed towards people in the front line, and the result of the approach is that it does not go beyond the attribution of blame. If a guilty person is found, he or she is held responsible for the accident. In practice this may well mean that the 'bad apple' is removed or punished. In fact, IBL is founded on a certain number of sound principles, beliefs that are valid for making choices and carrying out decisions. According to Reason [17], concern for the individual, typical of IBL, is based on some of the following beliefs: 1. Voluntarity of actions. People are considered as free agents capable of choosing between safe and unsafe behaviours. Numerous studies demonstrate that 80-90% of accidents involve human actions. Because such actions are perceived as subject to voluntary control, it is assumed that accidents are caused by negligence, inattention, inaccuracy, incompetence, etc. 2. Responsibility is personal. The personal model is founded on an assumption of individual responsibility. As in criminal law, the personal approach searches for the individual who is responsible for the error. 3. The sense of justice is strengthened. IBL is emotionally satisfying; after a serious accident, or worse, a disaster, the identification of blame tends to satisfy the people involved and the public in general. 4. Convenience. Conceiving of responsibility in terms of the individual undoubtedly has advantages for organisations from a legal and economic point of view, not least because it allows them to maintain unaltered their organisational structure, their rules and their power system. IBL is in line with the Western legal system. The goal of criminal law is to identify the individual responsible for a given event and to fix a punishment adequate for the type of crime committed. The search for the person responsible tends to direct an inquiry towards the identification of one or more people who committed the error. The people who directly provoke an accident are often the front line operators in the complex human–machine system. It is clearly easier to identify a person who is in close contact with the system (the pilot of a plane, the doctor, the nurse, the control panel operator, the train conductor, etc.) as responsible for the event, as opposed to the hidden, organisational and managerial factors which are the product of collective actions taken over the course of time. On the other hand, the individual blame logic brings with it a series of "perverse" or unwanted effects. In the first place, the identification of a guilty individual does not change the prevailing situation and does not improve the organisation. Secondly, the approach focuses on the past and creates a fear of legal disputes and sanctions, discouraging the reporting of errors on the part of front line operators and undermining the organisation's capacity to learn from them. Thus, IBL is not conducive to eliminating risk factors and does not guarantee that an analogous event will not reoccur with other actors. Finally, this approach is characterized by two particular forms of bias: *hindsight bias*[3] [18] and *fundamental attribution bias*[4] [19,20]. These factors make it difficult to openly discuss errors and to circulate information in relation to them, because the people involved fear that they will be blamed and that errors will continually be attributed to the personal inadequacies of individuals.

In reference to healthcare systems, Merry and Smith [21] declare that working under the threat of legal prosecution creates a climate of fear that is not conducive to the optimal use of staff in a medical system. Precisely for these reasons doctors tend to hide their errors and to engage in defensive medicine practices (the over-prescription of tests and treatments; avoiding high-risk procedures). The risk of losing face and the fear of legal disputes are powerful incentives for doctors to hide errors and engage in defensive behaviours. Goffman [22] states that "losing face" means feeling out of place or experiencing shame. If error – in itself involuntary – is viewed as an indication of professional incompetence and a source of possible legal prosecution, the propensity to hide it increases. The persistence of a blame culture, reinforced by a certain type of judicial action, becomes the principle obstacle to the creation of an effective culture of patient safety. A professional system, like that of medicine, that is subject to the constant risk of criminal investigation is not, then, a system that is more careful and attentive; rather, it is a system that reduces the risks of the people who operate within it by seeking greater formal guarantees of protection, thereby compromising the interests of the clients. Such is the origin of defensive medicine.

1.3. Defensive Medicine

Defensive medicine takes place when doctors, motivated primarily by the objective of reducing their exposure to medical malpractice litigation, prescribe unnecessary tests, procedures or specialist visits, or, alternatively, avoid patients or procedures that involve a high level of risk. When doctors engage in the excessive use of tests and procedures, they practice *positive defensive medicine*. When they avoid certain patients or procedures, they practice *negative defensive medicine* [23]. The increase in diagnostic uncertainty (tests, X-rays, etc.) influences in a significant way the practice of defensive medicine. The "defensive" use of technology has an avalanche effect: the more specialists prescribe unnecessary diagnostic procedures or aggressive treatments for low-risk situations, the more this type of approach becomes the new legal standard for clinical practice [24]. It is clear that all this has a great impact on healthcare costs and that it could contribute to a reduction in the quality of healthcare services:

---

[3] *Hindsight bias* has two distinguishing characteristics: 1) the "it was well known" notion, on account of which analysts emphasize what individuals ought to have known and prevented; 2) the lack of awareness of the influence that the knowledge of results exerts on the perception of past events. Thus, the facts appear straightforward and clear as opposed to ambiguous, contradictory and ill-defined, which is how they probably appeared to the actors at the time of the events themselves. Labeling a past action as erroneous is very often a judgment based on a distinct body of information available only after the event has taken place.

[4] *Fundamental attribution bias* is understood as the tendency that involves attributing blame for negative results to incompetence and inadequacy on the part of the actor in question as opposed to considering them as the product of a specific situation or as the result of situational factors beyond the control of the said actor.

unnecessary, invasive diagnostic procedures (for example, biopsies) represent useless risks for patients. Some estimates indicate that the practice of defensive medicine costs the American healthcare system in excess of $100 billion dollars annually, which would account for up to 12% of all healthcare expenditure [5]. As we shall see below, what has emerged in many countries, like the United States [25], seems to find confirmation also in the case of Italy.

1.3.1. Defensive Medicine in USA and Europe

While there has been considerable interest in the phenomenon of defensive medicine in the United States since as early as the 1960's, the interest in the rest of the world and Italy in particular is much more recent. As a consequence, while the literature on the subject in relation to Europe and the rest of the world is not particularly extensive, the literature in relation to the United States is vast. In 1978 Tancredi [26] identified a series of problem issues in respect of defensive medicine and assembled a wide range of evidence, concluding that about 70% of doctors engaged in defensive medicine practices out of a fear of malpractice litigation. In this epoch the Health Insurance Association of America estimated that the economic impact of defensive medicine was in the order of 3-6 million dollars per annum. In the 80's and 90's as many as 47 studies on the subject were conducted by research bodies or individual academics in the United States, some on a national level and others on a local level, some relating to the full range of specialities and others only to a subset of specialities or a single speciality [27]. A certain number of these studies sought to estimate the cost of defensive medicine. The most significant of the studies both in terms of their methodology and influence were those of Reynolds and Lewin-VHI [28]. Reynolds estimated that the total cost of defensive medicine for the year 1987 was 12 million dollars while for 1993 Lewin-VHI proposed a figure of 24 million dollars. In respect of the year 1992 the OTA [23] estimated that the cost of defensive medicine just in relation to complications associated with caesarean births was 8.7 million dollars, while its estimate in relation to head injuries in young people amounted to 44.7 million dollars. A study conducted by the Harvard Medical School Department of Health Policy and Management demonstrated that the majority of specialists in the various specialities adopt a "defensive" professional strategy [24]. The American researchers analysed a group of specialists operating in the specialities that were characterised by a higher level of litigation (emergency medicine, general surgery, orthopaedic surgery, neurosurgery, obstetrics and gynaecology and radiology). Out of a total of 824 doctors operating in 6 healthcare structures in Pennsylvania, 93% declared that they practised defensive medicine. In particular, 92% stated that they prescribed tests and procedures and made referrals readily, while 43% stated that they prescribed diagnostic procedures that were clinically unnecessary. Avoiding procedures and patients that are perceived as "dangerous" from a judicial point of view is another very widespread practice: 42% of the interviewees admitted that they had deliberately limited the scope of their professional activity so as to avoid complications. In 2006 Pricewaterhouse Coopers issued a report on waste in the American healthcare system, suggesting that the overall cost of waste was 1.2 trillion dollars per annum [29]. It identified three categories of avoidable costs: those consequent upon unhealthy behaviours like smoking, poor eating etc., those attributable to inefficient administrative procedures like the management of insurance claims etc. and those arising out of medical error, unnecessary hospitalisations, hospital infections and defensive medicine. It estimated that the cost of the latter category amounted to 210 million dollars. Using data from NAMCS (National Ambulatory Medical Care Survey), Merenstein [30] assessed the appropriateness of a sample of medical prescriptions by comparing the recorded justifications with the standards established by USPSTF (United States Preventive Services Task Force). Referring to a number of different types of prescriptions, he reported that the percentage of unnecessary prescriptions in the various categories ranged from 5% to 37% and estimated that the annual cost of these instances of waste varied from 47 to 194 million dollars. In a study of doctors operating in casualty departments in California between 2001 and 2005, Rodriguez [31] reported that about 50% declared that they were concerned about the issue of malpractice litigation. Analysing Medicare data on a range of serious illnesses in respect of the years 1984–87-89, Kessler and McClellan [32,33] – publishing in the prestigious review NBER (National Bureau of Economic Research) – reported that, while the most urgent need was for legislative reform in the area of reimbursements, the cost of defensive medicine amounted to 5 – 9% of overall expenditure.

Similar results emerged from a study conducted in Japan in 2006 [34] on a group of 131 gastroenterologists. 98% of the interviewees declared that they had practised defensive medicine and this was attributed to the increase in litigation. According to the researchers, the tendency of the doctors to effect an excessive number of tests and to avoid risky procedures is related as much as anything to the concern generated by the overexposure of the problem of malpractice in the media and by the consequential suspicious attitude on the part of the patient.

Academic interest in defensive medicine in Europe being more recent, the literature is not so extensive. Summerton reported a series of findings on the practice of defensive medicine in England [25,35]: 90% of doctors declared that because of a concern for medical litigation they dedicated to the drafting of patients' records a greater amount of time than they otherwise would; 86% stated that they furnished patients with explanations about procedures that were more detailed than would otherwise have been the case; and 40% indicated that they prescribed a greater number of screening tests than they otherwise would.

2. Methods

The object of the present study is to investigate the professional behaviour of doctors in Italy with a view to determining whether they practice defensive medicine and, if so, in what form and to what extent. In particular, in keeping with similar studies conducted in countries like the United States, Canada, Japan and Great Britain [24,25,34,36] a series of specific practices are identified - taking care to distinguish those representing positive defensive medicine from those typical of negative defensive medicine - and an attempt is made to represent their frequency in numerical terms. To carry out the study, the researchers developed a structured questionnaire composed of nine questions, divided into two areas:

1. The type of defensive behaviours most commonly adopted;
2. The reasons that induce doctors to resort to defensive medicine.

The study takes into consideration various forms of defensive medicine (prescriptions of drugs, referrals to specialists, diagnostic tests (laboratory and instrumental) and hospitalisations) and seeks to investigate the reasons that lie behind the choice to practice defensive medicine. In respect of this second objective it focuses on the following concerns of doctors: the fear of having to face litigation; the fear of receiving claims for compensation; and the fear of compromising their reputation and jeopardising their career.

The NS was conducted between July and November 2008 and involved 1,000 general practitioners, to whom the questionnaire was sent via e-mail. About 37% of the recipients (307 doctors) completed the questionnaire. The LS was conducted between October 2008 and January 2009 and involved 124 specialists, 60 anaesthetists and 64 surgeons, to whom the questionnaire was delivered by hand. In this case 82.2% of the recipients completed the questionnaire. The principle results are presented below.

3. Results

The doctors interviewed indicated that the problem of defensive medicine is becoming increasingly widespread. They stated that they frequently prescribe tests, treatments and specialist visits, or alternatively, avoid highly risky patients or procedures with the principle objective of avoiding exposure to accusations of malpractice.

3.1. The National Study (NS)

77.9% of the interviewees in the NS had practised at least one form of defensive medicine in the working month prior to being interviewed. The doctors most inclined to adopt defensive behaviours tend to be quite young. 92.3% of the interviewees in the 32 – 42 age bracket declared that they had practised at least one form of defensive medicine in the working month prior to the interview.

Table 2. Composition in percentage terms of the frequency with which defensive behaviors took place, broken down on the basis of the variable of "age" (NS)

	Frequency of defensive medicine behaviours during the previous working month		
Age	**Never**	**At least once**	**Total**
32-42	7.7	92.3	100.0
43-52	16.7	83.3	100.0
53-62	24.8	75.2	100.0
63-72	32.6	67.4	100.0

If we consider only the doctors that stated that they had engaged in conduct of a defensive kind (77.9%), we can see that the most widespread types of defensive behaviour are as follows (Table 3):

Table 3. Composition in percentage terms of responses to the question "In the course of the last month of work how many times did you perform the actions specified below?" (Aggregate data, NS)

	Never	From 1 to 6 times	From 7 to 10 or more times	Total
Prescribed a number of diagnostic tests greater than was necessary	38.7	53.0	8.3	100.0
Prescribed unnecessary invasive procedures (e.g. biopsies)	85.7	13.8	0.5	100.0
Prescribed unnecessary treatments	75.6	22.0	2.4	100.0
Prescribed drugs not strictly necessary	48.5	44.8	6.7	100.0
Acceded to/proposed the hospitalisation of a patient even though his/her condition would have permitted a surgery-based treatment	31.2	63.3	5.5	100.0
Made an unnecessary referral to a specialist	41.4	53.5	5.1	100.0
Wrote in a patient's records notes that he/she would not have written if he/she had not been concerned about possible future medical-legal problems	17.2	63.1	19.7	100.0
Avoided risky procedures on patients who might have been able to draw some benefit from them	86.0	14.0	0.0	100.0
Excluded "risky" patients from certain treatments	73.8	25.4	0.8	100.0

The following findings are of particular interest:

- the insertion into patients' records of otherwise superfluous notes was practised by 82.8% of interviewees;
- the proposal of hospitalisation for a patient that could have been managed otherwise was practised by 68.8% of interviewees;
- the prescription of a greater than necessary number of diagnostic tests was practised by 61.3% (A);
- the unnecessary consultation of specialists was practised by 58,6%;
- the prescription of unnecessary drugs was practised by 51,5%.

As far as the practice of *negative defensive medicine* is concerned, 26.2% of the interviewees declared that they had excluded from certain treatments patients subject to risk (i.e. beyond the dictates of a normal level of prudence). This figure, though inferior to those relating to positive defensive medicine, has an even greater importance to the extent that it relates to a form of behaviour that may well be subject to some form of litigation.

3.2. The Local Study (LS)

83.3% of the interviewees in the LS had practised at least one form of defensive medicine in the working month prior to being interviewed.

Table 4. Composition in percentage terms of the frequency with which defensive behaviors took place, broken down on the basis of the variable of "age" (LS)

	Frequency of defensive medicine behaviours during the previous working month		
Age	**Never**	**At least once**	**Total**
32-42	10.6	89.4	100.0
43-52	27.5	72.5	100.0
53-68	6.6	93.4	100.0

The most widespread types of defensive behaviour are as follows (Table 5):

Table 5. Composition in percentage terms of responses to the question "In the course of the last month of work how many times did you perform the actions specified below?" (Aggregate data, LS)

	Never	**From 1 to 6 times**	**From 7 to 10 or more times**	**Total**
Prescribed a number of diagnostic tests greater than was necessary	47	44.8	8.2	100.0
Prescribed unnecessary invasive procedures (e.g. biopsies)	95.3	4.7	0	100.0
Prescribed unnecessary treatments	65.8	30.7	3.5	100.0
Prescribed drugs not strictly necessary	42.3	49.5	8.2	100.0
Acceded to/proposed the hospitalisation of a patient even though his/her condition would have permitted a surgery-based treatment	69.5	28.2	2.3	100.0
Made an unnecessary referral to a specialist	51.7	41.3	7	100.0
Wrote in a patient's records notes that he/she would not have written if he/she had not been concerned about possible future medical-legal problems	21.1	56.6	22.3	100.0
Avoided risky procedures on patients who might have been able to draw some benefit from them	75.2	22.5	2.3	100.0
Excluded "risky" patients from certain treatments	73.1	25.8	1.1	100.0

The following findings are of particular interest:

- the most frequently adopted behaviour was the insertion into patients' records of otherwise superfluous notes. This was practised by 78.9% of interviewees;
- the prescription of unnecessary drugs was practised by 57.7%, the prescription of a greater than necessary number of diagnostic tests by 53% and the ordering of unnecessary referrals to specialists by 48.3%;
- the proposal of hospitalisation for a patient that could have been managed otherwise was practised by only 30.5% of interviewees;
- the least frequently adopted behaviour was the prescription of unnecessary invasive procedures. This was practised by only 4.7% of interviewees.

As far as the practice of *negative defensive medicine* is concerned, 26.9% of the interviewees declared that they had excluded from certain treatments patients subject to risk (i.e. beyond the dictates of a normal level of prudence).

If we break down the findings of the *LS* in terms of the two subsets of specialists interviewed – i.e. the surgeons and the anaesthetists – the results are quite different:

- the anesthetists revealed a more marked tendency to resort to defensive medicine. 88.3% of the anaesthetists declared that they had practised at least one form of defensive medicine in the previous month. The figure for the surgeons was 76.1% ;
- or both types of specialist, the most frequently adopted form of defensive medicine - as in the case of the *NS* – was the insertion into patients' records of otherwise superfluous notes;
- the practise of prescribing unnecessary drugs was more common among the anaesthetists than among the surgeons (64.2% as against 46.9%)
- the surgeons were characterised by a highly marked tendency to order the hospitalisation of patients who could be managed otherwise (62.5% as against a figure of 11.3% for anaesthetists).

From the data analyzed we can see, then, that the reasons that induce doctors to modify their behaviour during the course of medical practice relate principally to the concern that they will be sued for malpractice. In particular, in the NS the following results emerged (Table 6):

Table 6. The reasons for defensive behaviors (Aggregate data, NS)

What factors influenced of the behaviours indicated above?	**Agree**	**Disagree**	**Total**
1. Fear of a request for compensation	59.8	40.2	100.0
2. Fear medical-legal litigation	80.4	19.6	100.0
3. Fear of disciplinary sanctions	15.0	85.0	100.0
4. Fear of negative publicity, loss of image	43.5	56.5	100.0
5. Previous personal experience of medical-legal litigation	51.8	48.2	100.0
6. Previous experience of a colleague being subject to medical-legal litigation	65.7	34.3	100.0

Similar results emerged in the LS (Table7):

Table 7. The reasons for defensive behaviors (Aggregate data, LS)

What factors influenced the behaviours indicated above?	**Agree**	**Disagree**	**Total**
1. Fear of a request for compensation	67.1	32.9	100.0
2. Fear of medical-legal litigation	88.3	11.7	100.0
3. Fear of disciplinary sanctions	31.8	68.2	100.0
4. Fear of negative publicity, loss of image	29.5	70.5	100.0
5. Previous personal experience of medical-legal litigation	41.2	58.8	100.0
6. Previous experience of a colleague being subject to medical-legal litigation	68.3	31.7	100.0

The findings of the *LS* confirm that the fear of litigation is the major reason why doctors practise defensive medicine. So far as the different categories of specialists are concerned, the surgeons emerged as considerably more apprehensive than the anaesthetists. 75% of the surgeons declared that they had practiced defensive medicine because they had been afraid of receiving a request for compensation. The figure for the anaesthetists was 62.3%. 90.7% of the surgeons (as against 86.8% of the anaesthetists) stated that they had engaged in defensive medicine out of a fear of litigation, while 46.9% - and here the contrast with the figure for the anaesthetists (only 18.9%) is most marked – had done so out of fear of negative publicity or the loss of image. The findings indicate that the surgeons have significantly more direct contact with actual cases of litigation. 62.5% stated that they had had personal experience of litigation. The figure for anaesthetists was 28.4%. The same percentage of surgeons and anaesthetists declared that they had had experience of a colleague being subject to litigation.

4. Discussion

The results of the two studies indicate that Italian doctors – both general practitioners and surgeons – practice defensive medicine with a view to reducing the risk of being subject to litigation. In fact, Italian doctors frequently prescribe tests, treatments and specialist visits or, alternatively, avoid risky patients or procedures with the principle aim of reducing their exposure to accusations of malpractice. Moreover, the figures that emerged from the studies are of a magnitude comparable to that of those that have been published in studies on other countries. These results, then, confirm that in Italy, just as has already emerged in the United States, Japan and Great Britain, a significant number of healthcare workers modify their professional behaviour so as to protect their own career [24,34,36]. The exponential growth in patients' damages claims increases costs for both the public and private healthcare systems without leading to a corresponding increase either in the quality of the national healthcare system or patient safety.

The major conclusions that can be drawn from this study are:

11. *The existence of a high level of defensive medicine*. 77.9% of the general practitioners interviewed in the NS declared that they had practiced some form of defensive medicine in the working month prior to being interviewed. The percentage for the specialists interviewed in the LS was even higher: 83.3%. In addition, the findings of the LS suggest that in general anesthetists are more inclined to practice defensive medicine than surgeons. On the other hand, surgeons appear more inclined than anesthetists to order the hospitalization of patients that could be managed otherwise (62.5%) and to make referrals to other specialists.
12. *The fear of medical litigation*. 80% of the general practitioners of the NS who adopted a defensive approach indicated that they feared that they would be involved in a legal dispute, while 60% declared that they feared that they would receive a damages claim. In the LS too the fear of medical-legal

litigation emerged as the principle factor determining the practice of defensive medicine on the part of specialists. In particular, surgeons appear more concerned than anaesthetists both about requests for compensation (75% as against 62.3%) and about medical-legal litigation (90.7% as against 86.8%)

13. *The fear of negative publicity*. A substantial component of the general practitioners interviewed in the NS (43.5%) expressed concern about the accusatory approach adopted by the media. In the LS the surgeons revealed a particularly marked fear of negative publicity and the loss of image.

The increase in doctor-patient legal disputes and related insurance costs forms part of a broader tendency that involves other people working in high-risk professions (air traffic controllers, pilots, etc). The emergence of a "consciousness of risk" has led society at large to demand increasingly higher levels of safety in respect of an increasingly larger number of sources and types of risk. The individual blame logic, oriented more towards the identification of a guilty individual as opposed to the key underlying circumstances that led to the error, may be considered to be among the major factors that have led to the spread of defensive medical practices in doctors. According to Benn Healey and Hollnagel [37], "to improve patient safety, healthcare organizations must move from a retrospective focus upon adverse events to more proactive improvement processes that actively anticipate and mitigate vulnerabilities inherent in the system". Healthcare must develop the capacity to learn from errors and system failures and become more resilient and reliable. Resilient organizations [38] are those that successfully detect dangerous conditions and adapt to absorb variations before serious harmful consequences arise [39]. To achieve this, a profound cultural transformation is required. In fact, the search for the guilty individual discourages the reporting of errors, making it difficult to learn from failures and promoting the spread of defensive behaviours.

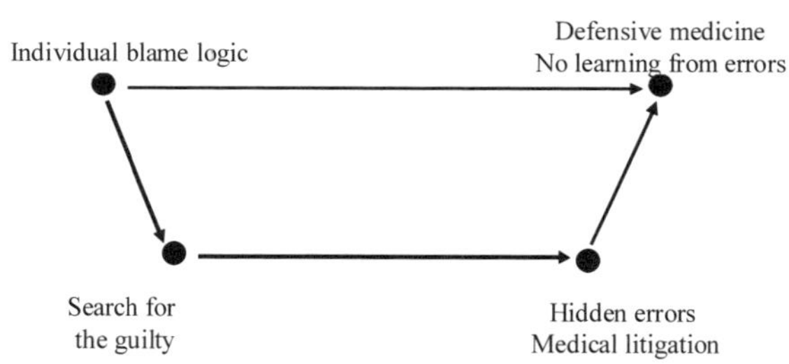

Figure 1. The mechanism that produces defensive medicine [14]

5. Conclusion

The two studies presented in this paper confirm that the phenomenon of defensive medicine is constantly increasing in Italy as it is in other countries. Moreover, they demonstrate that it is manifest both in the behavior of individual general practitioners working in relative autonomy and in the practice of specialists operating in a more integrated manner within the hospital system itself. This increase in defensive medicine is caused by the substantial increase in malpractice medical litigation. A punitive approach to error in hospitals encourages the phenomenon of defensive medicine and acts as an obstacle to the detection and reporting of error. To promote the visibility of errors and near misses it is necessary, on the one hand, to have more extensive and reliable information on accidents and, on the other, to create a certain number of "spaces of non-punishability" within which operators feel free to openly discuss failures so as to be able to learn from them. It must be recognized, however, that a completely non-blame organization runs the risk of lending approval to all unsafe actions. An organizational culture in which the scope of personal discretion is such as to render any type of action possible loses credibility in the eyes of the very people that operate in it [40]. A prerequisite for a fair and just safety culture is that all the members of an organization can identify the dividing line between unacceptable behaviors that merit sanctions and other behaviors in respect of which punishment does not help to promote safety. According to Amalberti et al. [41] the dominant values underlying medical practice (autonomy, craftsmanship) are in conflict with such safety values in critical ways. This conflict of values is the central threat to the achievement of ultra-safe healthcare. The findings presented in this article throw light on a further factor – the blame culture – which is shown to be a significant obstacle to promoting the detection and reporting of errors and to encouraging organizational learning to improve patient safety [14,42]. According to Jones [43] in the day-to-day reality of the hospital environment, certain cultural factors exacerbate/reinforce and expand/reinforce and extend the risks related to adverse events. To change these conditions, a profound cultural transformation is required. This cultural shift has to begin at the top of the organization in order for it to result in a positive effect on the behaviours of all organization members.

Finally, it is evident that it is necessary to rethink the use of criminal law, promoting a different civic epistemology [44] in the case of accidents caused by unintentional errors. Penal sanctions are clearly an important instrument for the social control of organizations but it is very doubtful – and, in fact, there is very little supporting empirical evidence – that they constitute an effective deterrent in the case of accidents [45,46] or that the recourse to criminal law can effectively prevent technological accidents like medical errors in the future.

The individual blame logic does not improve patient safety and it results in an increase in medical litigation and costs. There are good reasons to carefully evaluate the possibility of creating "spaces of non-punishability" within organizations like healthcare systems so as to reduce defensive medicine and to promote a process of learning from errors. It is to be hoped that such organizations benefit in the future from the promotion of a just culture [17,40,47] or, in other words, a culture in which front-line operators are not punished for actions, omissions or choices consistent with the level of experience they have but rather only for acts of gross negligence, violations or destructive actions viewed as intolerable.

The findings presented in this paper illustrate the importance of empirical research into the field of healthcare provision. In particular, the results demonstrate the utility of a research methodology that seeks to define clearly a set of concrete problem issues and to generate in relation to them readily interpretable numerical data. It is self-evident that the particular issue confronted in this paper – i.e. defensive medicine – has immense importance for healthcare systems, impacting, in particular, on the health of patients, the costs of healthcare provision and the organisation of the healthcare system. The findings that have emerged from the present paper already contain interesting suggestions for policy in respect of all three areas. Further empirical research can only serve to render these suggestions clearer and in the long term make provision for informed and carefully guided improvements to healthcare services.

References

[1] European Commission, Medical Errors, Special Eurobarometer 241 (2006), Bruxelles, European Commission.
[2] Kohn LT, Corrigan JM and Donaldson MS (2000), To err is human. Building a Safer Health System. National Academy Press,Washington.
[3] Vincent C (2005), The Evolution of patient safety. Communication at the International Conference on Healthcare Systems, Ergonomics and Patient Safety, Florence (Italy): 30/03/05-02/04/05.
[4] De Vries EN, Ramrattan MA, Smorenburg SM, Gouma DJ and Boermeester MA (2008), The incidence and nature of in-hospital adverse events: a systematic review. Qual. Saf. Health Care, 17: 216-223.
[5] Tillinghast-Towers Perrin (2003), U.S. Tort Costs: 2003 Update, Trends and Findings on the Cost of the U.S. Tort System 17.
[6] Ania (2007), L'assicurazione italiana 2006/2007. This can be downloaded from: http: //www.ania.it/ documenti_salastampa/convegni/82_199_03072007_con.pdf.
[7] Charles S. et al (1984), Physicians' self reports of reactions to malpractice litigation. American Journal of Psychiatry, 141: 563-65.
[8] Charles S et al (1985), Sued and non-sued physicians' self reported reaction to malpractice litigation. American Journal of Psychiatry, 142: 437-40.
[9] Maeve E. and Charles V (1994), The effects of medical accidents and litigation on doctors and patients. Law and Policy, 16: 97-121
[10] Committee on professional liability (2001), Coping with stress of malpractice Litigation. Journal of Gynecological Obstetrics,: 74: 65-66.
[11] Fileni, A. et al (2007), Malpractice stress syndrome in radiologists and radiotherapists: perceived causes and consequences. La Radiologia Medica: 112: 1069-1084.
[12] Law S (1986), A consumer perspective on medical malpractice. Law and contemporary problems, 49: 305-320.
[13] Elmore J (2005), Does litigation influence medical practice? Radiology, 236: 37-46.
[14] Catino M. (2008), A Review of Literature: Individual Blame vs. Organizational Function Logics in Accident Analysis. Journal of Contingencies and Crisis Management, 16, 1: 53-62.
[15] Avery RD and Ivancevich JM (1980), Punishment in Organizations: A Review, Propositions, and Research Suggestions. Academy of Management Review, 5: 123–132.
[16] Helsloot I (2007), Beyond Symbolism: on the Need for a Rational Perspective on Crisis Management. Boom Juridische Uitgevers, The Hague, Netherlands.
[17] Reason J (1997), Managing Risk: Organizational Accidents. Ashegate, Aldershot.
[18] Fischoff B (1975), Hindsight * foresight: the effect of outcome knowledge on judgment under uncertainty. Journal of Experimental Psychology: Human Perception and Performance, 1(3): 288-299.
[19] Fiske ST and Taylor SE (1984), Social Cognition. Random House, New York, NY.
[20] Gilbert DT and Malone PS (1995), The correspondence bias. Psychological Bulletin, 117: 21-38.
[21] Merry A and Smith AMC (2001), Errors, Medicine and the Law. Cambridge University Press, Cambridge.
[22] Goffman E (1963), Stigma: notes on the Management of Spoiled Identity. Simon & Schuster.
[23] US Congress, Office of Technology Assessment (1994), Defensive medicine and medical malpractice. OTA – H – 602, DC: US Government Printing Office, Washington.
[24] Studdert DM, Mello MM, Sage WM, DesRoches CM, Peugh JMA, Zapert K and Brennan TA (2005), Defensive medicine among high-risk specialist physicians in a volatile malpractice environment. JAMA, 293: 2609-2617
[25] Summerton N (1995), Positive and negative factors in defensive medicine: a questionnaire study of general practitioners. BMJ, 310(6988): 1200
[26] Tancredi LR and Barondess JA (1978), The problem of defensive medicine. Science, 200: 879-82.
[27] Baldwin LM, Hart LG, Lloyd M, Fordyce M and Rosenblatt RA (1995), Defensive medicine and obstetrics. JAMA, 274: 1606-10.
[28] Lewin-VHI (1997), Estimating the costs of defensive medicine. Report prepared for the MMI Companies, Va, Fairfax, January.
[29] Pricewaterhouse Coopers (2006), The Price of excess. USA.
[30] Merenstein D et al (2006), Use and costs of non recommended tests during routine preventive health exams. American Journal of Preventive Medicine, 30: 521-27.
[31] Rodriguez, R. et al (2007), A longitudinal study of emergency medicine. Academic of Emergency Medicine,: 14.
[32] Kessler DP and McClellan M (1996), Do doctors practice defensive medicine? Quarterly Journal of Economics, 111: 353-90.

[33] Kessler, D and McClellan M (1996), Do doctors practice defensive medicine? National Bureau of Economic Research, working paper 5466.
[34] Hiyama T, Yoshihara M, Tanaka S, Urabe Y, Ikegami Y, Fukuhara T and Chayama K (2006), Defensive medicine practices among gastroenterologists in Japan. World J Gastroenterol., 21-12(47): 7671-5.
[35] Summerton N (2000), Trends in negative defensive medicine within general practice. Br. J. Gen. Pract., 50(456): 565-6.
[36] Passmore K and Leung WC (2002), Defensive practice among psychiatrists: a questionnaire survey. Postgrad. Med. J., 78: 671–673.
[37] Benn J, Heakey AN and Hollnagel E (2008), Improving performance in surgical systems. Cognition, Technology & Work, 10, N. 4.: 323-333.
[38] Hollnagel E, Woods DD and Leveson N (2006), Resilience engineering: concepts and precepts. Ashgate, Aldershot.
[39] Patterson ES, Woods DD, Cook RI, Render ML and Bogner (2005) Collaborative cross-checking to enhance resilience. Paper presented at the 49th annual meeting of the Human Factors and Ergonomics Society.
[40] Reason J (1998), Achieving a safe culture: theory and practice. Work & Stress, 12, 3: 293-306.
[41] Amalberti R, Auroy Y, Berwick D and Barach P (2005), Five system barriers to achieving ultrasafe health care. Ann Intern Med, 142: 756-764.
[42] Catino M and Albolino S (2007) Learning from Failures. The role of No-Blame Culture, paper presented at 23rd EGOS Colloquium, Vienna, 5-7 July.
[43] Jones B (2002), Nurses and the "Code of Silence". In Rosenthal M. M. and Sutcliffe K. M. (Eds) Medical Errors. What Do We Know, What Do We Do. Jossey Bass, S. Francisco: 84-100.
[44] Jasanoff S (2005), Restoring Reason: Causal Narratives and Political Culture. In Hutter B, Power M Organizational Encounters with Risks. Cambridge University Press, Cambridge, UK.
[45] Vaughan D (1998), Rational Choice, Situate Action, and the Social Control of Organizations. Law and Society Review, 32: 23-61.
[46] Vaughan D (1996), The Challenger Launch Decision. Risk Technology, Culture, and Deviance at NASA. The University Chicago Press, Chicago.
[47] Dekker S (2007), Just Culture: Balancing Safety and Accountability. Ashgate Publishing Limited, Aldershot.

Detection and Prevention of Adverse Drug Events
R. Beuscart et al. (Eds.)
IOS Press, 2009

Subject Index

Author Index